S0-BXM-305

For my friend Amy
who is always motivated
to become a better
human being

Sandra Torres

LOSE WEIGHT PERMANENTLY

EFFECTIVE BODY TRANSFORMATION THROUGH LIFESTYLE CHANGES

Sandro Torres Cigarroa

authorHOUSE®

AuthorHouse™
1663 Liberty Drive
Bloomington, IN 47403
www.authorhouse.com
Phone: 1 (800) 839-8640

© 2015 Sandro Torres Cigarroa. All rights reserved.

No part of this book may be reproduced, stored in a retrieval system, or transmitted by any means without the written permission of the author.

Published by AuthorHouse 08/11/2015

ISBN: 978-1-5049-1791-9 (sc)
ISBN: 978-1-5049-1790-2 (e)

Library of Congress Control Number: 2015911088

Print information available on the last page.

Any people depicted in stock imagery provided by Thinkstock are models, and such images are being used for illustrative purposes only.
Certain stock imagery © Thinkstock.

This book is printed on acid-free paper.

Because of the dynamic nature of the Internet, any web addresses or links contained in this book may have changed since publication and may no longer be valid. The views expressed in this work are solely those of the author and do not necessarily reflect the views of the publisher, and the publisher hereby disclaims any responsibility for them.

Contents

Introduction

One of the things that has helped me overcome difficult times and achieve my goals is examining people's case studies and testimonials. Real people who have struggled to overcome difficulties in life like to help others overcome theirs. In addition, people who have overcome a negative habit know from experience, not by theory, how to help an individual who is going through the same difficulty. For example, a rehabbed alcoholic knows the steps necessary to overcome the bad habit of drinking. He or she knows the denial stage, the anger stage, and so on. This person has lived through rehabilitation and has valuable insight into how another will react to the process. Therefore, it is easier for a rehabbed person to help other alcoholics than it is for someone who has only learned the theory. Rehabbed people also know that helping others can help them stay sober. This could be one of the reasons that recovered alcoholics are so passionate about helping other alcoholics. They have made a commitment with themselves and a Superior Power to help others. People who have overcome difficulties such as obesity, alcoholism, mental disorders, or drug addiction leave instructions to help others rehabilitate. They leave testimonials, how-to steps, self-help books, articles, and so on.

This book is based on true stories and true people. However, the names have been replaced by fictitious ones to protect the privacy of the individuals. Although this self-help book is written in novel form to keep the reader entertained, the goal of the book is more than entertainment. Its goals are: to help the reader to lose weight permanently; to have a healthy lifestyle, healthy body weight, and healthy mind and by the end to find true happiness. The concepts presented here have been applied by people who have been successful in reaching their goals.

I would like you to take your life and this book seriously in order to change your life. Albert Einstein said, "Any man who reads too much and uses his own brain too little falls into lazy habits of thinking." Consider the information provided and see if it makes sense to you. If you question any of it, do your own research until you find the truth that can help you achieve your weight loss goals.

About the Author

Sandro Torres is the founder and owner of Custom Body Fitness, a training studio in Carbondale, Colorado, that specializes in weight loss and body transformation. Sandro is certified by the American Council on Exercise as a personal trainer, life coach, and weight management specialist. He is also the secretary of board of directors of a local community health center. Sandro is studying psychology, and he loves to learn. Therefore, he reads books by different authors whose insights and information have contributed to this book. After all, we all learn from each other and explain our information in our own way.

After suffering a significant loss, Sandro fell into depression. He found positive ways to overcome this mental state, and he then understood that the only way to achieve happiness is by helping others. Since then, Sandro has worked with the purpose of helping those who want to be helped and who are ready to change their lives.

Sandro is the founder and owner of Custom Body Fitness LLC located in Carbondale, Colorado. He is a certified life coach, weight management specialist, and personal trainer certified by ACE.

Sandro Torres Cigarroa

Sandro was born in Mexico City in 1981 and move to Carbondale in 2000. He went back to college in 2010 and founded Custom Body Fitness the same year. His business is a local success.

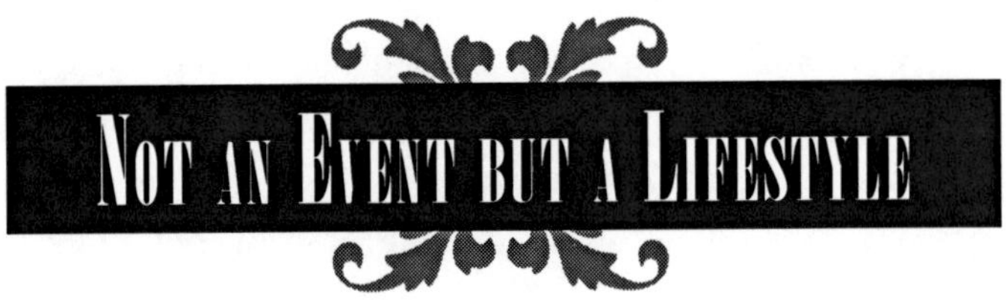

Not an Event but a Lifestyle

"I want to see fast results."
"Tell me why you want to see fast results."
"Because I'm tired of feeling tired, not feeling good about my body, and having this extra weight. I'm also tired of the doctor repeatedly telling me to lose weight because of my diabetes."
"So you think that by losing weight fast, all these concerns will go away?"
"Yes."
"Weight loss is not an event but a lifestyle. So the real problem is not your weight, but the life you live."

This is how we began Mary's weight-loss program. Like many other clients, Mary did not have any knowledge about weight loss. She had a distorted perception about weight loss. She believed in many myths, products that promised fast results, diets that were by no means healthy, and risky hormones and medical procedures that carry health risks. I knew we were about to start a long journey. My only concern was if she was ready. I knew I was ready. I remembered the words of Lao-Tzu: "A journey of a thousand miles begins with the first step." So we started with the first step, a conversation to explore her goals, her ideas, and her willingness to make crucial changes in her life.

Mary wanted to hear that her problems would disappear with her weight loss, but she didn't realize the opposite was true: *her weight would disappear when she took care of her problems.* She asked, "What do you mean by 'not an event but a lifestyle'?"

"Here, let me explain," I started. "The situation that troubles you—your lack of energy, not feeling good about your body, and your susceptibility to diabetes—is not because of the extra weight you carry. It is because of your lifestyle. The extra weight you carry is due to your lifestyle as well. The habits you have developed throughout your life are the ones that have put you where you are." I knew that the research done by Omichinski in 2010 backed me up, so I added, "There is plenty of research on this. Not everyone who is overweight develops diabetes, and not everyone who has diabetes is overweight. Once again, the deciding factor is their lifestyle."

I could see that she was paying close attention to what I said. "What about how I feel?" she asked.

I was happy to see that I had sparked her interest. I replied, "As with many things, several factors contribute to how people feel. Yes, your appearance and your extra weight do contribute to some degree to how you feel. However, don't forget that we can find people who have a healthy weight or are even underweight who still feel like they need to lose weight. Environment, feedback, traumas, and other people also contribute to one's self-esteem." I paused and smiled. "But let's not deviate from the subject. Yes, I can help you lose weight. If losing weight fast is what you are looking for, I can give you a recommended eating plan and an extreme exercise regimen where you will spend more than fifteen hours a week exercising, where all you can think about is exercise and following the meal plan. If you follow this step by step, you will lose weight, Mary, I promise. But what is the point? Are you going to do this for life? Can you keep it up? Are you going to enjoy it? Or does it just sound like something you *have* to do?"

She looked down, and I could see a moment of contemplation. "But I can lose the weight I want to lose and then just change my life, right?" she asked.

"Maybe. People tend to avoid the difficult path and find shortcuts. This is the reason promising diets and pills are so popular," I responded. "People want everything easy and fast. The reality is that what's going to help you lose weight is not the event but the habits that you are changing. Do your own research. According to an online article I read by Lauren Lopez, studies show that nearly 95 percent of people fail to achieve their weight-loss goal, and 95 percent of the 5 percent who lose weight regain it. This means that out of a group of four hundred people, 380 will quit their weight-loss program. So that leaves twenty people who successfully lose weight for the first months and years. Out of these twenty, nineteen will regain their weight. So this leaves us with one successful person who loses weight permanently. Four hundred people try and one succeeds. Why did the other 399 fail? They didn't focus on their lives; they focused on the event. They don't understand that the solution is within them, not the regimen they followed. Also keep in mind that many of these people already know the steps to follow to accomplish weight loss: exercise and healthy eating. Then why don't most people succeed?

"According to the American Council on Exercise, one of the largest and most trusted organizations in this field, weight problems involve a complex interaction of many factors involving psychological, environmental, evolutionary, biological, and genetic causes. In other words, for many people, making healthier food choices is not as easy as it seems it should be. Our psychological barriers from past experiences make us choose auto-destructive behaviors such as overeating. People are stressed by the environment, and many people see value in areas other than the good habits they have developed. We are evolving to a fast-paced life in which material things seem to be more valuable than our health. Our body is biologically made to be active, but when compared to our ancestors, we have become dangerously sedentary. They did everything with physical effort, including hunting, farming, childcare, and even protecting themselves from predators. Now our most difficult task is putting the clothes in the laundry; the rest of the time we sit in front of the TV or a computer, stand around at our jobs, or just sit at a desk. For most of us, physical activity is not required in our working environment. In addition, because we are eating foods that make us fat, our genes are becoming weaker to these foods and, therefore, we are fatter," I explained.

"I think what you are telling me is interesting, but I need specific objectives. How should I start?" Mary asked.

"You should start by identifying your bad habits and replacing them with good habits," I answered. "That is what I teach and how I can help you be successful in your weight-loss program. Once you lose the weight, it is gone forever. You won't be regaining what you lose."

"So where should I start? Mary asked.

I smiled. "Since you are here, I'm guessing that you understand that you are signing up for an exercise program. That makes me think that you are ready to be active," I said.

"Yes, but I also need help with my diet. Do you provide assistance in dieting as well?" Mary asked.

"Yes," I replied. "We are going to help you change your eating habits but not get you on a specific diet. Our plan requires more than an exercise program for success. Let me tell you what we are going to help you with. You are going to learn about positive and negative habits, about myths such as BMI—the scale, fat levels, and predispositions—foods, scheduling, emotional eating, and what fits your lifestyle, because not everyone is the same. You'll also learn about emotions that affect your body, meditation as stress management, priorities and managing your day to fit all you need to do in one day, and, of course, exercise—how it affects the body, what you should do, what are the best exercises, and how they help. We will educate you about food to answer your question."

"Sounds good, now how many times do I need to come to exercise?" Mary asked.

"Here at the studio only three or four times," I answered.

"But I'm not sure if I would be able to make it. I'm so busy with work, my family, and school," she said.

"Well, Mary, let me ask you this: how important is your health? Do you want to lose weight, feel great, have more energy, and not develop diabetes?" I asked.

"Yes, I want all that."

"Why?"

"Because I want to live longer. I want to be healthier, I want to play with my children, and I want to look and feel good."

"Is that all?"

"What else do you want to hear?" she asked.

"I want to hear the conclusion. I'm going to tell you the real reason: you want to be happy. This is the reason human beings exist, and this is why we do what we do—to be happy. So if you don't start now and don't get rid of bad habits now, you will never reach your goal. Guess what? You are *always* going to be busy. Now there are your children, work, and school. Later, it will be your business or your work again, your grandchildren, and your deteriorating health, which you can minimize starting now. I've found that when people say, 'I'll do it tomorrow, next week, next month, or next year,' it just never happens," I told her.

"You are right. I have wanted to lose weight for at least five years, and I never have the time. Now that I think about, I have been busy since I became independent. I opt for easy ways out; *shortcuts* is how you described them," she explained.

Mary is a twenty-nine-year-old woman who is five feet two inches tall and weighs 192 pounds with 38 percent fat levels (fat levels taken with an electromagnetic impedance machine). There were no skinfold measurements, since her fat levels were too high for the skinfold caliper. Her circumference measurements by inches were as follows:

Neck: 12.10
Upper Arm: 13.08

Chest: 40
Waist: 35.02
Abdomen: 36.04
Hips: 49
Thigh: 30.04
Calf: 16.06

I told Mary that she could achieve anything she wanted to and explained that the only limitations were those she created. We finished the first assessment (goals, barriers, mental stage, and medical history), and we were very happy to begin her weight-loss program.

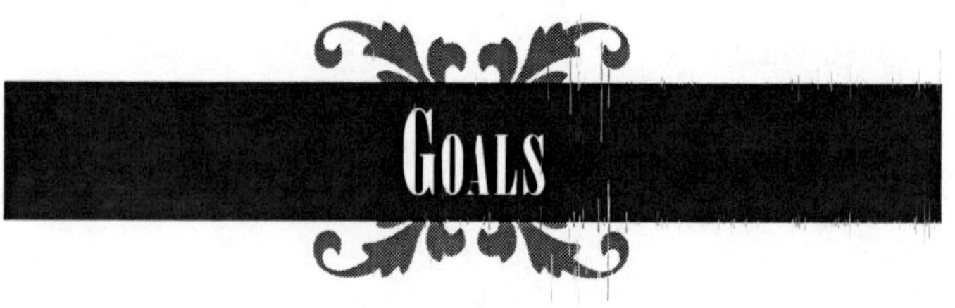

Goals

It was a cloudy Saturday. It looked like it could rain any minute. I had planned to hike a thirteen-thousand-foot mountain. Hiking is one of my favorite activities. It helps me clear my mind and ask deep questions about my life. As I was hiking, I asked myself why many people are successful in their weight loss and others are not. Even though there are many factors, I discovered that goal setting is very important. Many instinctively grasp the concept, while others must learn the behavior. I came up with a simple example to illustrate goal setting—about when I wanted to buy my first car, which cost me only three thousand dollars. I had a clear idea of the car I wanted, who I was going to buy it from, and how much I wanted to pay for it. I did not have the money collected yet. My brain started to calculate how many more hours I needed to work, and how much money was needed for the car payment, insurance, gasoline, and repairs. It sounds silly, but that is how goal-setting works.

I stopped to contemplate this thirteen-thousand-foot mountain. I felt some water drops, but I decided to continue my hike. I kept thinking, and this led me to another question. Why is it so difficult for some people to achieve an ideal weight? Well, a material thing—such as a car—is tangible. In contrast, one's dream body isn't. Also, it is not so difficult to get a car; people work, save money, find a car, and buy it. Simple. On the other hand, to reach an ideal weight, people need to pay for services, struggle with emotions, be able to see the value in what they're doing, break intangible barriers, engage in physical activity that they are not used to, and make an overall change in their lives. They don't get it in one easy exchange, like buying a car. Their bodies change gradually; the process is slow.

I read it over and over again. Goal setting is the key. People who are successful in weight loss, business, and family relationships know this, and they follow the same pattern. Goals need to be specific, measurable, accountable, realistic, and time bound. The voice of Mary's voice got into my head: *My goals for this month are to lose weight, eat healthy, and exercise. I want to be able to run. I want to change my life.* I was halfway up the mountain and the rain was pouring, so I decided to hide under a tree until the rain calmed down a little. The Rocky Mountains have capricious weather. So as I waited out the storm, I continued my line of thought. All of Mary's goals are good, but they weren't specific. They needed to be specific. She needed to see them clearly, touch them, smell them, and taste them. It reminded me of the story of the Asian master from the book, *The Monk Who Sold His Ferrari*:

> *Near where we were sitting there was a magnificent oak tree. The sage pulled one of the roses from the garland he habitually wore and placed it on the centerof the trunk.*
>
> *Yogi Raman then asked Julian to put the handkerchief over his eyes as a blindfold.*

"How far from the rose am I?" Yogi Raman asked his pupil.

"One hundred feet," Julian guessed.
"Have you ever observed me in my daily practice of this ancient sport of archery?"

"I have seen you strike the bull's-eye from a mark almost three hundred feet away, and I cannot recall a time that you have ever missed at your current distance," Julian noted dutifully.

Then, with his eyes covered by the cloth and his feet placed securely on the earth, the teacher drew the bow with all his energy and released the arrow—aiming directly at the rose hanging from the tree. The arrow struck the large oak with a thud, missing its mark by an embarrassingly large distance.

"I thought you were going to display more of your magical abilities, Yogi Raman. What happened?"

"Today's demonstration is meant to reinforce my advice on the importance of setting clearly defined objectives in your life and knowing precisely where you are going. What you just saw confirms the most important principle for anyone seeking to attain their goals and to fulfill their life's purpose: you will never be able to hit a target that you cannot see."

The rain stopped, and I could see the blue sky and hear the birds singing again. I told Mary to *specify* her goals for her weight loss, healthy eating, and exercise habits—as well as what running meant to her and the behaviors she wanted to change in her life. After exchanging ideas we found some *realistic* goals. I still remember what she said: *I got it, so I'm losing between three to six pounds of fat this month. To get there, I'm starting to eat my breakfast, snack, lunch, and dinner; to buy organic; to avoid drinks with added sugar, to drink only water; and to stop buying processed foods. I'm exercising three times a week from 5 to 6 p.m. every Monday, Wednesday, and Friday with a trainer, and I'm walking and jogging or hiking Tuesdays and Thursdays at 7 a.m. for thirty minutes. These are changes that I'm making in my life to feel better."* She had been happy with this clarification. She could touch her goals now and think about them. I remember reminding her that those goals were *time bound, measurable, and accountable* and that she needed to review and change her goals according to her lifestyle.

That sheet I provided her had a system in which she could clarify her goals in different areas, such as eating habits, eating schedule, stress, medication, weight lifting, cardiovascular training, and recreational activities. The sheet was divided into long- and short-term goals. When people set realistic and reliable goals, it is very possible to get there. Mary said that her goal was to lose forty-two pounds or to be on the 20 percent fitness category. So, we brainstormed about what would be possible. A person may lose from zero to twelve pounds a month. To be realistic, however, I recommend from one to eight pounds at month. Mary decided to set her goal for three to six pounds per month to be at her weight in seven to twelve months. Her percentage was 38 percent, and I have seeing people lose from nothing to 3 percent. We decided to use this percentage system rather than pounds. If she were to lose 1 to 2 percent a month, it would take her from nine to eighteen months to get to her goal. She told me that made sense.

I continued my hike to the top. I thought about my own goals during my hike. I read that people need to give themselves at least ten minutes to imagine their goals—that first the ideas are created in the brain, and then they will be manifested in the material world. There was no doubt that setting goals helped me in my journey in life. Setting goals is a skill that people need to master to succeed in losing weight. The hike was fun, and it was more than just exercise; it allowed me to meditate on the concept of goal-setting.

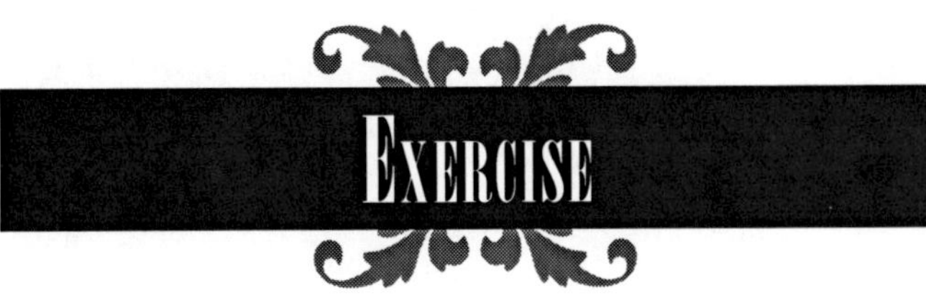

EXERCISE

"Hello, everyone. Welcome back."

This is how I began my 6 a.m. session on Wednesday. "Many people have a mental barrier, and they don't see beyond what they know. Here is an example: If a person has lifted only five, eight, and twelve pounds and has never been introduced to a heavier weight for any reason, they don't even know that fifteen pounds exists, or if they do, they consider it beyond their reach. It is very important that you challenge your body. Always look ahead and look for the next level. This is the only way to get results," I explained. "The body adapts to a new resistance. So if your goal is to lose weight, increase your metabolism, and be fit, you should overload your muscles. Overloading your muscles to the next level and continuing to safely increase the weight is called *periodization*. Periodization increases your muscle mass, which is called hypertrophy, and hypertrophic muscles require more calories, which increases your metabolism. In contrast, when you have a sedentary lifestyle, your muscles also adapt to the lack of resistance and will atrophy, burning fewer calories and decreasing your metabolism."

After these words, my team and I showed the routine of the day, and everyone started exercising. The session was fun! All the participants gave their best in the training session. They showed their desire to change—not by words but by actions. When the session finished, Mary asked me, "So I should be lifting heavy all the time? I heard that high repetitions and lower weight is better than low repetitions and heavy weights."

"Muscles are made to do both, so you can do high and low repetitions," I explained. "Muscle strength is defined as one's ability to perform a single repetition with maximum resistance. Muscle endurance is one's ability to perform many repetitions with a sub maximum resistance High repetitions and low repetitions are correlated. The heaver you go with weights, the more strength you gain. This will help you do more repetitions with lighter weights. People can perform about ten repetitions with 75 percent of their maximum resistance. For example, if you can do one chest press repetition with twenty-pounders, then you may be able to do ten repetitions with fifteen-pounders. However, I don't recommend low repetitions as few as six because of the high risk of injury, but people can still do it. In addition, there are two main muscle fibers, slow-twitch and fast-twitch. When you do high repetition, you work the low-twitch muscle fibers: And when you do low repetitions, you work the fast-twitch muscle fibers. The reason I'm telling you this is because you need to work both muscle fibers, slow and fast. Neither one is better than the other. If you do only high repetitions, most likely you are training only the slow-twitch muscle fibers, and usually people who do high reps don't even use enough resistance. So you're better off running than doing this type of training."

"But I don't want to get bulky," Mary said.

She was referring to one of the popular myths many women believe. Some people believe things that they don't actually understand, and they don't make an effort to do their own research. They believe what others have to say or what society believes. I don't blame them. I used to be in the same wagon. So I replied, "First you have to take into consideration hormone levels. According to the American Council on Exercise, a high-resistance training program (six to ten repetitions) will usually lead to significant hypertrophy in most males. Most females, because of naturally lower levels of testosterone, will not generate significant hypertrophy even with this type of program. This does not mean that you won't tone your muscles. You will increase your muscle mass but not to a point where you look like a man. You will have your feminine body with the difference that your body will show muscle tone. Let me explain; testosterone is what makes a man a man. In other words, we have high levels of testosterone compared to women. You, in contrast, have 90 to 95 percent less than what we have; You may find this information at Sharecare.com. Testosterone is the reason men burn fat faster, and it's also why they develop big muscles. A normal woman with normal levels of testosterone—and I have never heard of a woman with the same levels of testosterone as a man—can't be as muscular as a man. There are some exceptions of women who are strong because of their physiology, such as muscle attachment, but that is another story. Your body most likely won't be able to do this, but if it does, you may stop any time before you reach that weight."

Mary was pleased with my explanation. She smiled and replied, "I can see all the before–and-afters and testimonials from all the people you helped. I trust you."

A month passed since Mary first began training with me, and it was time for her assessment. As an experienced trainer, I have noticed that not many people are excited about being assessed, and not everyone yields the same results. This is due to the following factors: the effort people put into exercise, changes to their eating habits, the time they've been carrying the extra weight, support from their peers, stress, medical issues, and beliefs. Some people have the belief that they can eat anything since they are exercising. The truth is that there is no program that can overcome a bad diet. Others believe that they are destined to be overweight. Also, some people's bodies need to adapt when put under a new stress, so the body does not respond by losing weight in the beginning. Honestly, I don't know what to expect from any of my clients in their second assessment. Some of them have lost up to fifteen pounds on the scale, while others gain five pounds in their second assessment. Those who don't focus on the scale and who concentrate on changing their bad habits see results faster than those who are focused on the scale.

Contrary to my belief, Mary was excited to be assessed and find her progression. She had given her best effort at her training sessions. She gave me the notebook where she had written her goals and had been tracking them. She had written: *I'm losing between three and six pounds of fat this month. To get there, I'm starting to eat my breakfast, snack, lunch, and dinner; to buy organic; to avoid drinks with added sugar, to drink only water; and to stop buying processed foods. I'm exercising three times a week from 5 to 6 p.m. every Monday, Wednesday, and Friday with a trainer, and I'm walking and jogging or hiking Tuesdays and Thursdays at 7 a.m. for thirty minutes."* In her notebook she had something like the following log:

Exercise Log

-Walking -Running -Swimming -Biking -Hiking -Strength Training -Other

Date	*Days*	*Activity/Time*	*Activity/Time*	*Activity/Time*	*Activity/Time*
	Monday	*Weights/1 hour*	*Run/30 mins*	*Dog Walk/40 mins*	
	Tuesday	*Run/1 hour*	*Dog walk/20 mins*		
	Wednesday	*Weights/1 hour*			
	Thursday	*Hike/40 mins*			
	Friday	*Weights/1 hour*	*Hike/40 mins*	*Dog walk/20 mins*	
	Saturday	*Weights/1 hour*			
	Sunday				

I'm grocery shopping every Saturday to have all I need to cook during the week. I'm buying all organic and have cut my television bill to afford the extra cost.

Breakfast: oatmeal made with water and raisins; or bowl of fruit: pineapple, cantaloupe, watermelon, grapes and 1/4 of cup of granola; or smoothie made with frozen fruits, parsley, kale and celery.

Snacks: an apple, or a pear, or a banana, or baby carrots, or two oranges, or three peaches

Lunch: Leftovers from last night's dinner; wheat bread sandwich made with avocado, sprouts, cream cheese, tomatoes, onions, roasted veggies, and roasted mushrooms

Dinner: Chicken stew made with all types of veggies including zucchini, squash, broccoli, Brussels sprouts, cauliflower, carrots; make organic wheat pasta with the same veggies; pan fry veggies with steamed rice.

Mary told me that she was referring to her goal sheet to cook based on what she had decided. She also said that she would change some things, and she gave me an example: "Instead of chicken, I would use beef." Mary still had many questions about weight training, so she asked, "How is weight lifting helping me lose weight? Why not stick with running and healthy eating?"

"Running and healthy eating will help you lose weight, no doubt," I answered. "But keep in mind that cardiovascular training such as running cannot be replaced by weight lifting nor weight lifting by cardiovascular training. Same with eating healthy eating. It can't be replaced by exercising only. Weight lifting will give you many benefits that other types of training won't, such as strengthening your muscles, ligaments, tendons, and bones. This will help you prevent injuries and also will help you to lift more weight, which will allow you to burn more calories and also will increase your metabolism. In a proper program with the right intensity you will burn up to eight hundred calories in fifty minutes in your training. Cardiovascular training has a limitation on muscle development because of the range of motion and the resistance put into the muscle. Let's take running into consideration. Your knees don't bend ninety degrees when you are running, so some muscle fibers do no work as compared to lunges, for instance. When you are running, you are not carrying a forty-five-pound weight, either. Running is about the intensity of the exercise, not resistance. To expect to build lots of muscle from running is like wanting to get toned with light weights and high repetitions; it's the same concept. Running is also is a high-impact exercise; it is already stressing various joints including the knees. If you were willing to put a forty-five-pound weight on your back when running, you'd be putting your knees and other joints at risk of injury. This is the reason that running is not recommended for overweight people," I explained.

I paused and then said, "I'm only guessing that you not only want to lose weight, but you also want to have a great appearance. Cardiovascular training helps you lose weight, but it won't tone your muscles if you have no muscles to tone. Plus, as I mentioned before, it won't give you the strength to lift something heavier than you are used to. Keep in mind that the body starts aging after twenty-six years of age. What this means is that the human body starts losing 5 percent of muscle mass every decade for both males and females. This is normal. Weight training will aid you by building new muscle fibers to counter what aging is taking from you. So the lose areas that you feel in your body are nothing other than accumulated fat, no muscle. Your muscle mass is gone, and you need to put it back on. As you do, the fat will diminish, and the muscle will tone. In addition, your body goes into a process called remodeling, which happens every seven years. What this progress does is disintegrate your bone mass and rebuild it. If you don't stress your bone mass by exercising—weight lifting, for example—the new bone structure will be weaker the next time it rebuilds itself, and this is one factor that leads to bone weakness or osteoporosis. Cardiovascular training also plays a big role in aging. When the body ages, the stroke volume decreases. Stroke volume is the amount of blood that the heart sends through the body each time it beats. The blood does many things, such as cleaning up waste from our bodies, healing the body, delivering oxygen, nourishing tissues, and many other things. So if there is not enough blood traveling through the body, the body is not as efficient. And I forgot to tell you, burning calories is a chemical reaction between fat and oxygen or carbohydrates and oxygen. Exercise rejuvenates your body, burns calories, and clears up your mind—among other benefits that food can't replace. So you can lose weight doing only one habit, but it won't be optimum weight loss." I looked at her and asked her, "Did that answer your question?"

"Yes," she answered, "but are you telling me that the body's normal process of aging makes us fat, weaker, and less efficient?"

"If you put it that way, yes. However, exercise slows down the process of aging."

"So exercise rejuvenates the body and makes it function like when I was twenty years of age?"

"More or less," I answered with a smile.

"You recommended that I should come to train here three to four days and to do cardiovascular training at least three times a week. Why?" Mary asked.

The American College of Sports Medicine recommends that adults should do some type of strength training two to three times a week to gain some muscle. I recommend three to four times a week of weight training and at least two days of cardiovascular training. I have noticed a lot of change in my clients in three months with these recommendations."

"Okay, can I do strength training five to six days a week?" Mary asked.

"I really don't have a specific answer," I told her. "But I can tell you what I have found out."

I noticed that Mary was really interested and ready to lose weight. However, my concern was whether she was ready to change her life to keep the weight off. Many people who are desperate to lose weight are willing to overtrain, and typically they can't maintain the effort in the future.

"Research shows that people who overtrain lose motivation, feel tired, are susceptible to injury, have a weak immune system, and are more likely to drop their fitness program. Also I have found out with my clients that they suffer from pain in the knees and lower back. Plus, they don't do their best when they are training five times a week and they get sick more frequently," I explained. "Keep in mind that weight loss is a lifestyle, and I'd guess that you also have other priorities in life. Find a balance, and you will enjoy your weight-loss program."

"If I find a balance, I would be enjoying other areas of my life, and I will be looking forward to exercise. But I want to lose weight fast," Mary said.

"I know that," I said. "Most people want the same, just as most people want to become rich overnight. Many people are talented or win the lottery, but they have not developed the habits of a millionaire. Same thing happens with your body. Many people want an athletic or healthy body, but they do not understand the terms athletic or healthy. The body is only a reflection of the habits. An athlete is a person who is good at sports or any physical exercise. To accomplish this, the athlete must train. Healthy is a synonym for *well*. Well means *good*, and what creates a healthy body are good habits."

Mary was open to new information. Something inside her was telling her that she was doing well. She would get impatient like many people, however. Patience is a virtue that people develop. Just like Mary was doing her best to be patient, I had to model the same by being patient with Mary.

I took Mary's measurements; she weighed 181 pounds, and her fat percentage went down to 36 percent measured with the bioelectronics impedance. Her circumference measurements now were as follows:

Neck: 12.06
Upper Arm: 12.14
Chest: 38.12
Waist: 30.10
Abdominal: 33.12
Hips: 46.12
Thigh: 28.04
Calf: 16

We needed to talk about the next habit since she was doing well with exercise and eating. So I mentioned it. "Do you meditate?" I asked.

She responded with no hesitation, "No, I don't."

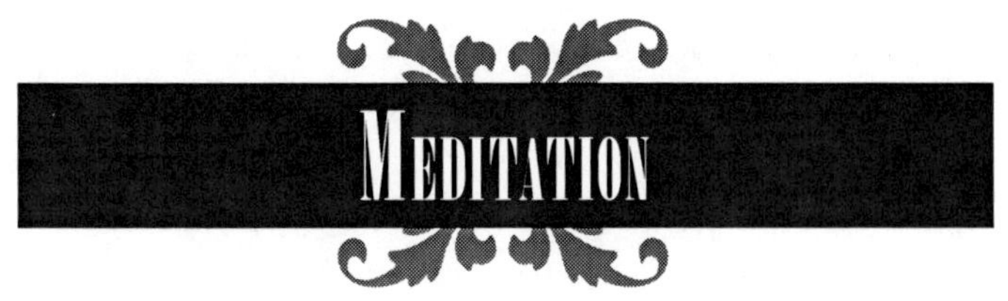

Meditation

"One of the most important things we can do is meditate, because meditation is a process that causes the brain to function as it's designed to, using both the left and right hemispheres in the proper way. I read this in a book called *Power Thoughts* by Joyce Meyers. Keep in mind that you don't have to believe that everything I have said is true. When a professional comes and gives you information, you should consider it critically. I might just want to persuade you to do something that benefits me. You can't be sure if the professional is looking at you as the dollar sign or if he or she really cares about you. Also, he or she can be persuaded by other organizations and might not even have accurate information. The only way you can find the truth is through meditation. My words are nothing more than information, and you will never understand the deep meaning until you meditate on them."

I continued telling her the benefits of meditation. "Meditation will help you with stress.

When you gather information and meditate about your past, you will be able to understand many unresolved issues. Therefore, you will be able to forgive yourself and others. Forgiveness will release you from negative feelings and by the end will help you with your weight loss. Forgiveness is practiced only by superior people, and meditation helps with this process. People who forgive know that if they do so, they have less chance of falling into autodestructive behaviors. When you meditate about the present and consider all the options for the decisions you need to make, you will know what you want, and the environment won't be able to influence you. For example, if you are thinking about buying fast food because you saw a commercial that got you all fired up about the taste, price, and convenience, you can step back and think about if you really want it, if it's healthy, if it will harm your health, or if you're even hungry. So the environment is the commercial, but you are getting it out of your head by meditating."

I had explained why Mary should meditate about the past and present. Now I needed to encourage to her to meditate about her future. "When you meditate about the future, you will know what steps to take to prevent things from happening that you don't want to happen. You'll also be able to get what you want from life. Sometimes people are confused about their feelings. They don't understand that their feelings are a product of their thoughts, so when people meditate about their thoughts, they identify their thoughts, and they control their feelings. Here are four ways I meditate:

1. As I walk and read, I think about the my past, my mistakes, my successes, and what is either bothering me at the moment or making me smile. Like anyone else, you are human, and you are allowed to make mistakes. However, these mistakes are not productive if you try to avoid dealing with them.

The best thing you can do is meditate on them to find an answer or solution. Answers will help you understand the outcome of your decisions, which in turn will help you make better decisions in the future. In other words, you study your past to not make the same mistakes—or to improve your outcome. Solutions will help you fix the past. For example, if you stole something, you may want to return it. Or, if you conclude that you need to ask for forgiveness, be brave, call the person, and ask. What will probably happen is that the other person will recognize his or her mistakes, and you two can find a solution. When you are noble, the rest will follow. Any mistake that you made in the past can be avoid in the future if you meditate about it, and you will feel better when you fix your mistakes.

2. I kneel down and give thanks for everything I have and have gone through, even those moments that I think are not good. I thank God for another day, for having my family, for the economic status I have, for the cars, the house, the food, the struggles, my business, my knowledge, my success, my body, my sight, my hearing, and so on.
3. I sit, cross my legs, interlace my fingers, and close my eyes. I picture myself in the future as a successful person in the area in which I want to be successful. For anything to be realized it first needs to be created in the mind.
4. Information is always coming into my life. Anything I read, hear, or see—I then process and study to determine if it's fact or fiction. Meditating

on this information helps me find reality and get closer to my goal. What I call the *environment* is everything that is outside of us, and sometimes the environment can have a negative effect on people. Perhaps a car salesman in a commercial convinces you that a new car is the key to your happiness or the solution to your problems, so you buy one that you don't need or can't afford. Another example is when people tell you that what you want to achieve is impossible. Though you should believe in yourself, they have convinced you that you can't do it. Here is where *I* define what I want from life and myself, not what the environment wants from me. To feel even more strongly about my decisions, I reinforce my mind with good information. Here is an example: If someone comes and tells you that you are wasting your time trying to lose weight because you are not going to change, you may believe that. But you have the ability to get those words out of your head, read articles that support what you want to accomplish, and keep going in your journey, because you know inside that you will change. You have the power to change your destiny, and meditation plays a big role," I said. Mary was quietly listening like a patient student whose teacher was explaining what to study to get the right grade on the final exam.

"I never thought about it that way," she replied. "I thought meditation was only making your mind quiet and blank and humming like a weirdo. So I might already be meditating sometimes when I wash my dishes or cook.

When my husband takes the kids to the park while I cook, I turn the TV off and do my chores silently. This is when I make the best conclusions about the decisionsI make in my life. Now that I'm cooking more often, I'm making better decisions in life, including in my weight-loss program. Is thinking when I'm cooking like meditating?"

"Absolutely," I responded. "If there are no distractions, such as other people, music, television, or anything else that interferes with your thoughts and cooking. So you are doing well. Now I want you to continue meditating, but just like any other habit, do it consistently, every day for at least twenty minutes. You can even do it when you are hiking or running. Just remember the requirements: no music, friends, cellphone, or other distractions that can take your focus from your thoughts."

Mary added one more goal to her goal sheet: to continue following all the steps to lose six pounds of fat this time. She was happy that she had exceeded her goal of six pounds by two pounds, which put her at eight pounds off. Then she asked, "What else can I do to continue with my goals?"

"I think you are rocking!" I said. "It is okay to add only one habit a month if you continue following the good habits that you set up last month. Some people struggle and can't follow their first month's goals, and, therefore, they don't get results. They get discouraged and they relapse. And the cycle starts again. But you are following through. Continue with those habits and your goals, make them a lifestyle, and don't forget to find a balance. Exercise and eating healthy is just part of your life, not your life. Enjoy your family, work, hobbies, and personal growth.

Mary gave a huge smile. She was very happy with her assessment and ready to start the next month.

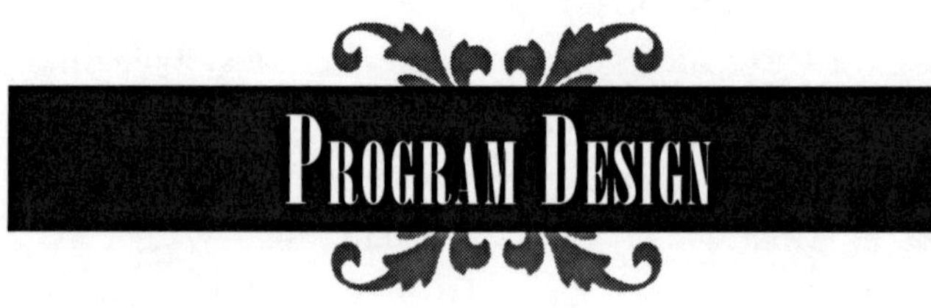

Mary and I had developed a great friendship. She was letting me help her, and I was teaching her the steps to succeed in her weight-loss goals. The best thing about Mary was that she was like a child when it comes to learning; she was open-minded and curious. She had many questions. The problem with many adults is that they think they know everything, and it can be hard to teach them new ideas. But Mary was just enjoying her journey and learning. In her second month of training, she was going away to visit her parents. Because she was seeing good results and feeling great, Mary wanted to continue exercising while she was away. The idea of trying other training sessions was not very appealing to her. She loved the training she'd been following. Even though I told her to just stay active and run, hike, and take a break from weight training, she wanted to continue lifting. It's true that a week or two-week break after six months or more of weight lifting is beneficial; it allows the body to heal, and the mental rest can lead to an enthusiastic return to training. But it was only her second month, so I decided to help her design a program, because that's what she requested.

"I'm leaving this coming Monday for two weeks," she said. "Can I get my program designed before then, so I can take it with me?"

"Because you don't have any injuries or limitations, such as knee or heart problems, it will be easy to design a program for you," I answered. "I'll do it this week, and I will make sure it is in your inbox by Monday. I'll probably design your program with basic exercises, so you can perform them with confidence. What do you think?"

"Yes, it's fine with me. Just make sure I get it. I don't want to be lazy on my vacation."

The following Thursday morning I started working on Mary's program design. I needed to include some important instructions even though she had heard them from me before.

Hello Mary,

I hope you are having a great trip. Here is what I promised, your program design. Also, I'm going to remind you about a couple of pointers for performing your exercises correctly. Please feel free to e-mail me if you have any additional questions.

- *Your posture is very important, so make sure you are using the right form at all times. Don't lift weights just for lifting. You need to know the right form, of which you have an idea by now. If you are not sure, check some videos online or send me an e-mail back, so I can further explain the exercise.*
- *Make sure you progress and continue lifting heavier weights as your body allows you to. Here is an example: If you curl ten-pound dumbbells and they become easy to curl, then you want to curl twelve-pound dumbbells. And when the twelves become easy, use fifteens and so*

on. This is called periodization. So, continue lifting safely even though I'm not around.

- *You should target all the big muscle groups in the body, such as the quadriceps, hamstrings, core, pectorals, back, triceps, biceps, and shoulders. This will allow you to be strong like a chain. The chain is only as strong as its weakest link. This means that if you have strong arms but weak legs or core, you might injure yourself. Plus, you may create a muscle imbalance—by working only your chest but not your back, for example. Also, working your whole body will help you have a better body appearance. I'm responsible for designing a complete body exercise program, but the reason I'm giving you all this information is so you finish the entire program and don't just drop it halfway.*

Many program designs work. They are like cars—there is one for every taste and need. This one is designed for healthy people who want to lose weight and tone their bodies, so they can follow this program with no problem.

Warm up:

Run, bike, or do some other cardiovascular activity for six to ten minutes. You can also do the following:

Jumping jacks for one minute, mountain climbers for one minute, jump rope for one minute; then repeat the sequence two times.

Once you are warmed up, you may begin doing the program. Make sure you rest one minute between exercise sequences.

First sequence:

- *10 push-ups*
- *20 alternative lunges*
- *20 double crunches*
- *1 minute jumping jacks*
- *Rest 1 minute*

Repeat the sequence three times.

- *10 inverted pull-ups*
- *10 Romanian death lifts*
- *20 alternative curls*
- *1 minute mountain climbers*
- *Rest 1 minute*

Repeat the sequence three times.

- *10 overhead triceps extensions*
- *10 military press*
- *1 minute plank*
- *I minute jump rope*
- *Rest 1 minute*

Repeat the sequence three times.

To cool down, develop a series of appropriate stretches for five to ten minutes.

> *There you have it, Mary. These exercises are pretty basic with low risk injury. You can follow this program three to four times a week, as you have been doing here. Remember that soreness is a reminder that you just had an awesome workout! It will also remind you that you are getting closer to your goal. You stressed the muscles enough to create microscopic tears in them. They will heal, make*

> *you stronger, and get you in shape. Remember to continue your running and healthy eating habits, because no training can overcome a bad diet. Enjoy your vacation, and I'm looking forward to seeing you back at the training studio.*

I finished the e-mail and sent it to her. I was so proud of her that she was making exercise part of her life. Not many people want to exercise on their vacation; only those who are committed to their goals are willing to exercise even on their vacation.

Priorities and Planning

A priority is something that is more important than other things, yet sometimes people make trivial things a priority. When I interview some of my clients, they don't have a clear understanding of priorities. Some people were raised in a chaotic way and were never taught how to prioritize their lives. As adults, they still prioritize trivial behaviors unconsciously. I thought about how important it is to prioritize behaviors in life, so I decided to write a newsletter about priorities.

Priorities and planning are very important for achieving a healthy body weight and living a healthy life. There are 24 hours in one day and one night. Planning the day and focusing on one's priorities make the day more efficient and productive, helping you to reach a goal, such as losing weight or maintaining an ideal weight. This way, trivial things such as watching television get pushed to the side. What really matters is what is going to contribute positively to your life. It is like an investment that will yield profit in the future. Think about what really matters at the end of the day. What is going to add up to make your life better? What do you really care about and what is more valuable to you in general? Let me give you an example. My priorities are my purpose, my family, my health, my education, my financial status, and lastly, my hobbies.

My purpose is what motivates me to wake up and continue my life. My purpose gives sense to my life. To be more specific, to help others every day and positively change this world is what I look for every day.

To me, family is everything. I don't think it's worth fighting for anything else if I don't fight for my family. And habits are thought first at the family relations. Once the family gets corrupted, the world follows.

My life depends on my health. If I were sick, I would not be productive and focused on my purpose, and I wouldn't be able to perform to my potential.

Education is what I need to continue teaching, understand myself and others, and give the right information to those I help.

Money is what the world usually uses to exchange services and products. I don't see money as my ultimate goal but as a tool to continue helping others without stress.

And my hobbies are practices that help me stay fresh and are things that I enjoy.

Can you see how my priorities are clear and it's logical why I made them a priority? Now I will express how I put my priorities into practice.

My focus is to make a difference in this world by helping both my clients and organizations that protect and fight for what I believe in. Also, giving value to the world is part of my purpose. This is a priority at which I work every day at my business. This is what I have in my head when I train my clients and write.

My family is part of my life. Changing the world is caring about others, and if I care about others, I care deeply about my family. So fighting to make this world a better place begins with the family. I spend weekends with my brother, and almost every night we cook dinner and enjoy our time together. I do my best to listen to him and help him become enlightened. I work on our relationship every day.

My health depends on many habits that I practice during the day, including having an eating schedule, eating the right foods, learning about nutrition, meditating, and exercising. I have my breakfast, snacks, lunch, and dinner scheduled. I buy organic when I go shopping and invest my money there instead of other products such as alcohol that will harm my health. I exercise every day no matter what. And I walk every day to meditate.

Sometimes I take college classes or renew my certifications. The information might be valuable, but personally I think schools have an agenda and usually teach theories in general. Therefore, I continue my research by reading articles and books and making my own mistakes, studies, and conclusions. I like to try things out and practice after I gather information. So every day I read a book or article that interests me.

My hobbies are my breaks on the weekends. I enjoy working on my car, learning to play the guitar, learning to shoot a bow, and dancing. But I do not do any of these until all my other priorities are met.

These priorities take most of my day, but they contribute positively to my life. These priorities are positive habits that make my life fulfilling and healthier and make me happier. If you noticed, I have not made any destructive habits a priority, because they get pushed out of my life. My priorities come before any trivial things such as hanging out with negative people, watching TV, playing video games, surfing online, gossiping, shopping … and the list goes on.

So if you are looking for an ideal body weight, habits that contribute to your main goal should be priorities.

Committed to your happiness and well-being,

Sandro Torres

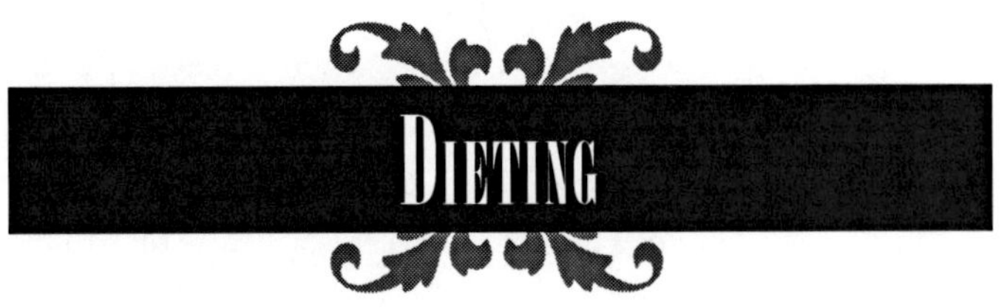

DIETING

Mary returned from her two weeks away. She was very excited about being back and continuing with her training. "How was your vacation?" I asked.

"It was great," she responded while she was getting her shoes tied to start training. "I feel refreshed and ready to continue with my goals even though I did the program that you sent me."

"Thank you for being so committed." I said to welcome her, and I started leading the session.

The training session was full with fifteen members. Two new members were waiting for instructions to start the sessions. The rest were talking about things they have in common.

After one hour of training, the session went well. Everyone pushed their bodies to their limits except for one member who was having a hard day. "Is everything okay?" I asked John.

"Yes, but it's hard for me today."

"It's okay, John. Everyone has those hard days. You did well. You pushed, and you are here. Many people don't show up when they have difficult days, but you made it. It is not okay to come and just *try* to train and waste your time. But what you did is what you could do. I can see it. So don't be hard on yourself. Tomorrow will be another day, and you will do better," I said winking at him.

"You're right; I just don't like it when it feels hard and takes more out of me. I feel like I'm not progressing. But I know what you're talking about, and I made it."

You are strong not because of your physical strength but because of your mind strength. We shook hands, and he signed up for his next sessions. Julie was next to sign up, but she wanted to talk to me. Therefore, I signed up everyone else first so Julie and I could have some privacy.

"What can I do for you, Julie?"

"I'm not getting the results I want," Julie said with a complaining tone of voice, like an unhappy member who has done it all to get results.

"Let's find out why, since you exercise hard and usually don't miss a session," I said.

"Yes, I know that. I'm following your exercise suggestions. This is the reason why I'm here telling you that is not working for me."

"Okay, what about the rest of your habits, such as your eating habits?"

"I started this diet, the paleo diet. I got off track, but I'm going back to it."

"I thought you had your eating habit goals figured out."

"Yes, but I think this diet works. My friend lost ten pounds with this diet," Julie said.

"Okay, so how do you explain your results?"

"I told you—I slipped," she said.

"Did your friend keep off the weight she lost?"

"No, she regained some of it."

"So she was successful in her diet?"

"Yes."

"Then, regaining the weight is being successful?"

"No. I mean, *yes*," Julie answered.

"So you want to lose weight, so you can gain it back and get on the yo-yo cycle, so you end up weighing more than before you started dieting?" I asked, thinking of Omichinski's study published in 2010.

"No, I don't want that."

"So let me ask you again—is dieting a successful way to lose weight?"

"Well, it is if I follow the regimen," she answered.

"So are you planning to live your whole life dieting, restraining yourself from eating foods that you want and others that you need?"

"No, if you put it that way, no. I was thinking to do it only for a period of time until I got to my desired weight."

"And then what, if you can make it that long with this diet?" I asked.

"Go back to eating the way I was eating" she said.

"And regain the weight you lost?"

"No," she replied after thinking for a couple seconds.

"Did you ask how your friend felt when she was dieting?" I asked.

"No."

"Maybe you should pay attention to how dieting people look and feel. Usually I get testimonials from people who dieted in the past. They say they lose weight but feel tired; their bodies are still loose. Or when they wear small clothing, the fat hangs, they crave candies, and they look pale."

"Now that you mention it, she does not look healthy and energetic. I think you are right," July said.

"Well, I don't want to be right. I want to help you understand why dieting does not work. Diets are popular. A close friend is dieting, a coworker, a family member, a teacher, and the neighbor. They lose weight—five, ten, or twenty pounds—and four months later, they weigh more than before they started dieting. *Why* is the question? The reality is that dieting is an illusion, the relief that people see on the scale while they're actually not losing fat but are harming their bodies. Linda Omichinski explains that weight fluctuation and repeated dieting are the real contributors to heart diseases, obesity, inadequate nutrition, fatigue, weakness, and gallstones. In addition, Linda further explains that some other psychological negative effects include weight obsession, poor self-image, disordered eating patterns, disordered lifestyle, and an increased sense of failure. People who have been dieting are likely to be out of tune with their bodies and natural signals of hunger and fullness.

Also, Nutrition Dimension, the world's leading nutrition education organization, claims, that people on diets do not have a normal, healthy relationship with food and are, therefore, destined to fail in their quest to lose weight. They will, in fact, be more likely to gain more in the long-term. Self-control is what many people rely on with dieting. They want to be able to say *no* to the nutrients that dieting prohibits, even though their body craves such nutrients because they are essential for survival; other professionals have other effective ways to avoid troublesome foods. Doctor Phil, in his book, *The Ultimate Weight Loss Solution,* recommends finding other ways to cope with food, such as avoiding places where trouble foods are going to be—but not trying to use self-control. Many diets restrict some essential nutrient the body needs, such as carbohydrates. People have a negative relationship with carbohydrates due to the publicity of certain diets. Linda Omichinski, a registered dietitian, says that dieters are not accustomed to eating carbohydrates. They are not aware that by eating more protein and cutting back on carbohydrates, such as bread and pasta, they are actually setting themselves up to crave carbohydrates from other sources, such as cake and cookies. The lack of carbohydrates in the body causes a person to crave sweets as a quick resource for fuel. This can make people gain weight, since they overeat calories with sweets, such as cookies. If people eat enough carbohydrates, the body will crave fewer sweets. Remember that carbohydrates are energy that the body uses in everyday life, especially for high intensity exercises."

"I never saw it this way," she told me, disappointed.

"Let me add more information," I said. "I read that dieting is the beginning of psychological issues such as binge eating, bulimia nervosa, and anorexia nervosa. As I said before, dieting is not healthy for your body or your mind. Period. I understand that you want to lose weight rapidly," I continued, "but this is the reason people can't get to their healthy weight or desired body. They want to do it quickly without really studying the consequences of the bad behaviors they are practicing. You literally have to change your life. The good news is that you don't have to do it all at once. You learn how to do it step by step."

After processing the information, Julie replied, "I think this diet is what is making me eat sweets. I crave more cake, cookies, and candies than ever. And if you said that the body asks for the nutrients that we deny it, I think that is what my body is asking for. And I stopped eating these foods that I don't want to eat."

"So what do you think is the real answer to getting the results you want?" I asked.

"I think I need to work at my eating habits," she said.

"We talked about how important it is to change your eating habits for life. Do you remember that at your first assessment?

"Yes, I do. Can we sit and talk about it again? I think I need to understand what I need to do right to eat healthy."

"Yes, we can set up an assessment and see where you are with your goals, your body fat percentage, and habits."

Julie and I agreed on an assessment time. Assessments are important for everyone to see where they stand—to find out what they need to work on, to evaluate what is giving them results, to develop new goals, to continue breaking barriers, and to reacquaint themselves with relevant information. Some people are on top of their assessments because they want to see their results from training hard and changing their life habits. On the other hand, some people panic and don't look forward to being assessed because they know they have not paid the price to get the results they are looking for. Therefore, the results disappoint them. Usually these results leave the member with a bad perception of assessments in general. They blame the assessment while ignoring the real source of the problem. Some clients who are not afraid to confront reality and who did not do the work take these poor results as a wakeup call. They get on their feet and figure out their mistakes and continue with their journey, leading to good results by the next assessment.

Julie left the studio and I was so focused on listening to her that I didn't notice that Mary was listening to our conversation; I didn't notice that she was still in the training studio.

"I'm sorry," she said, approaching me. "I really didn't mean to listen to your conversation, but I was so interested about what you think about dieting that your conversation caught my attention."

"Don't be sorry," I replied, seeing the look in her eyes, "It was not your mistake. I should have taken Julie to my office or at least made sure that there was nobody at the studio before we started our conversation. Anyway, I'm guessing you stayed because you want to know more about the topic."

"Yes, I want to know about habits that people can adopt to lose weight. I have been able to get good results because I'm following your recommendations. But don't you think that my goals require dieting? To achieve them I have to restrain myself from eating certain foods."

"Let's compare," I said. "Dieting usually targets food types and tells you to get one or more out of your diet—usually fats, protein, or carbohydrates. For example, they cut out either meats, fruits, some vegetable such as potatoes, or fats such as oils. They discriminate carbohydrates in general, including refined sugars or sugars that are in fruits. Changing your eating habits does not discard a nutrient. You are allowed to eat everything in moderation.

Diets usually tell you what to eat with no concern for the consequences. They usually follow a regimen where some products or foods are allowed without moderation, such as meats or ultra-processed yogurts just because they are protein. This applies to other nutrients allowed in the diet as well.

When you change your eating habits, you choose what to eat. Eating real food with moderation helps your psychological well-being, and it's easier to stick to the changes you decided to make. Dieting usually does not discard the ultra-processed foods that contribute negatively to your health. Many diets allow you to eat packaged food if they don't fall into the category of nutrients that they claim contributes to being overweight. For example, in some diets you are allowed to eat low-fat yogurts without paying attention to the amount of processed sugars or chemicals that yogurt has. Once again, they focus on nutrients—not the product.

By changing your eating habits, you understand that any nutrient from whole foods is good, and you are allowed to eat it. But ultra-processed food is not food anymore, and you should avoid things that the human being is not designed to eat. People usually think about 'all or nothing' with dieting, which means they follow it 100 percent or they quit 100 percent. However, they think that diets will be short-lived, for some weeks or months. Most people gain back what they lost and more by thinking this way, because they can't keep up with the diet, and it messes with their mental health. Changing your eating habits means that you can give up, change, or improve wherever you are ready to give up, change, or improve—taking into consideration that you want to become better at your eating every day. Here you understand what is bad for your health and change it as you want."

"Tell me more," Mary requested.

"Do you cook?" I asked.

"Yes, and I find it difficult to cook, but now that I'm using less processed foods, I find myself cooking more. Nevertheless, I'm so busy in my life that I feel like I don't have the time. I have to work, clean my house, exercise, and take care of my family."

"Cooking is not usually mentioned when you are dieting. You should know that you are eating healthy by changing your habits to cooking. Do you watch TV?"

"Yes, I do, but that is my relaxation time," she objected.

"TV time is not really relaxation time. Do you think your health is a priority?"

"Yes, that's the reason I'm here."

"So I'm going to assume that you are willing to put your health before anything negative that doesn't contribute to your health."

She looked at me as if she were wondering what I was going to talk about next.

"You want to know more about habits, right?" I asked.

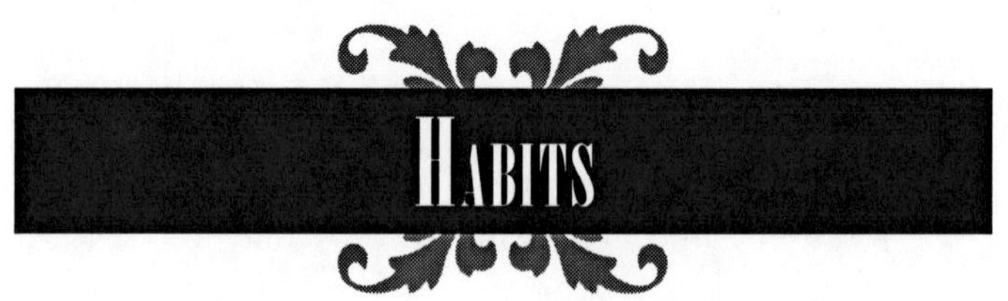

HABITS

"They are only two types of habits, negative and positive," I said. "Some people call them destructive and constructive habits, bad and good habits. People have both. Many authors emphasize the importance of changing bad habits for good habits. By the way, accourding to the authors of *The Power of Focus,* a habit is a behavior that people perform in their normal lives that becomes easier each time it's done, something that people repeat many times. Some habits we develop involve how we manage time or our finances, family traditions, and eating patterns. Good habits are hard to adopt because they require dedication, effort, and discipline. On the other hand, bad habits are easy to adopt because they do not require any dedication, effort, or discipline. Plus, they can make us feel short-term relief, but we do not pay attention to the long-term consequences. According to author Jack Canfield, 'Life does not just happen. Life is about choices as well as how to react to each situation. If you always make bad choices with frequency, disaster will happen.'

Since we want to focus on your dieting, we're going to talk about what you can do to accomplish your weight-loss goals by changing your eating habits. If you think about it and do some research, you'll see that different societies suffer from different problems. This is because of their habits. People do not gain weight overnight. Even a large baby did not gain the weight overnight. The mother makes a big contribution to the weight of her newborn baby. This contribution is not genetics but the habits of the family, especially the mother. Let me explain it by describing the *Dutch Hunger Affect* study: In 1944 the Nazis limited the food resources of people living in parts of the Netherlands. In this group of people were pregnant women who received only four hundred to eight hundred calories per day. The genes of the embryos responded to this environment by saving sugars and fats. Years later, when the embryos had grown to thirty- to forty-year-old adults and the food supply was back to normal, they suffered from heart problems such as high blood pressure and heart attacks. In other words, people are overweight because of the lifestyle they live—the bad habits. It's easier to blame it on genes and be blind to the reality than go the extra effort that it takes to stay healthy. In addition to this, keep in mind that people are distinguished by their habits. When someone wants to belong to a specific group of people, the first requirement is to develop the same habits of the group, even if they're negative habits—like drinking, eating at fast food restaurants, watching television, or being irresponsible. On the positive side, there are good habits, like cooking at home, reading, and exercising. If you keep this in mind, I think it's important to be very strict when picking the people that we spend time with. Now, let's conclude together what you can do to change your negative eating habits to good eating habits."

Mary was listening to me attentively, and she asked, "So people can change their physique?"

"Let me answer this question in a minute," I replied. "Do you want to lose the extra weight that you are carrying?"

"Yes, that's why I'm here."

"There is an easy way to do it."

"Tell me!" Mary asked me with excitement.

"Modeling."

When I talk to my clients, I lose the notion of time. I love teaching people what I have learned.

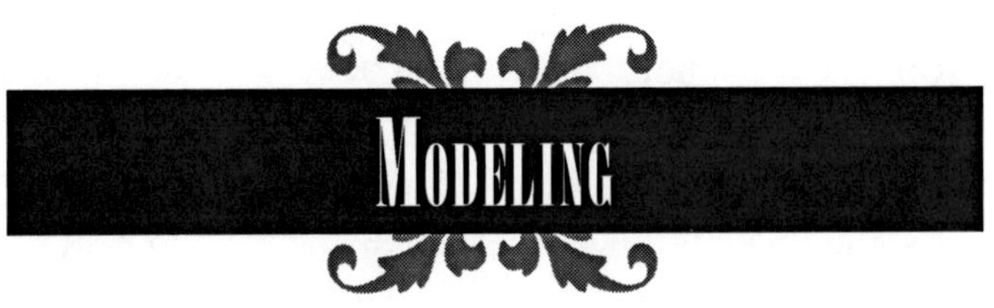

Modeling

"What do you mean by modeling? Oh, I know what that means," she responded right away. "If I get into modeling as a career, that will help me lose the extra pounds," she said, smiling sarcastically.

"No, imagine for a moment that there are no schools or educational institutions, and you want to learn how to swim, play the guitar, drive a car, or whatever. But you have friends who are very good at what you want to learn. What would you do?"

"Hang out with my friends so they can teach me," she answered.

"That is modeling. The same thing happens when you want to lose weight and reach your fitness goals. These people who know exactly what to do will teach all you need to know about weight loss. Now, remember that once you get there you need to maintain, and the best things you can do are modeling and finding a support group. Here is a testimonial from motivational speaker Anthony Robbins: 'I had produced the result of being extremely overweight. I began to realize that all I needed to do was model people who were thin, find out what they ate, how they ate, what they thought, and what their beliefs were, and I could produce the same results. Sounds easy enough? It is easy when you have the right support group or models to follow. Remember when we talked about getting rid of your 'crab' friends? Modeling people who are not crabs will lead you to success."

"But I don't know how to model," Mary said.

"You do know how to model. In fact, you do it all the time even though you are not conscious of it. Your behavior is due to the people whom you hang out with. We all model people, but some people model others unconsciously. Some people even model actors, actresses, or singers. The people whom we model the most are our family and peers." Look around and see who you act like. Or who acts like you. Of course, people do not imitate people, but people model others and somehow they do model the new behavior in their unique way. I do it all the time, even when I write. I know how to write because I read a lot. Other authors have taught me how to write and I model them own my own way."

"But I don't hang out with people who are active except for the people whom I met here."

"There you have the answer. You have to start hanging out with active people and model their lives, including their eating habits, to be able to get rid of those extra pounds. This is the easy way," I said with a wink.

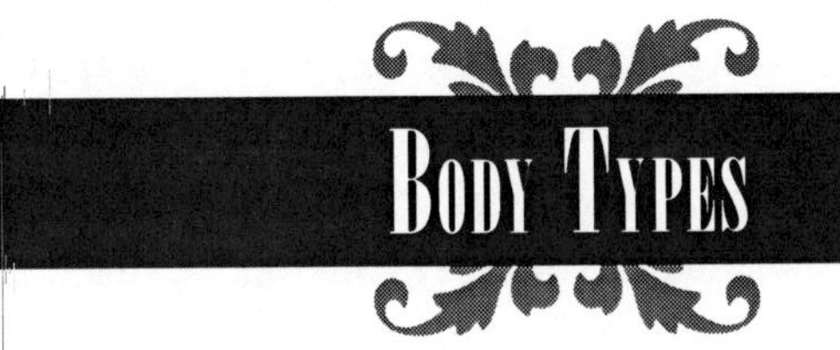

Body Types

"Getting back to the question you had earlier about whether people can change their physique: yes and no. Yes, because you can change the way your genes work by how you respond to the environment, meaning everything outside of yourself. For example, a person who is overweight because he or she eats the wrong foods, lives a sedentary lifestyle, drinks alcohol, or takes some medicines that contribute to obesity could make his genes respond differently by not practicing such behaviors. Usually people have a weakness; scientists call it predisposition, and religion calls it demons. The more a person stays away from those bad habits, the stronger the genes become. However, keep in mind that I'm not saying it's easy, and it does take mental and physical effort. The person who stops most of the destructive behaviors will develop a fit body. So people can change how their genes respond to the environment.

"So what about diseases that people claim to be genetic?"

"Many people do not understand the term *genetic*. When people think about genetics, they usually think that it is a predetermination and that there is nothing anyone can do to prevent diseases or change behaviors. The real definition of *genetic* is that there is a genetic contribution to the environment given to the gene. Therefore, the gene can be manipulated by the environment and thoughts as well. For example, a person who is predisposed to diabetes is not born with the disease, but his or her genes are susceptible to developing diabetes. That means that if the person lives a sedentary lifestyle (low insulin) and eats refined sugars (high sugar content), then chances are they will develop diabetes. However, if they don't practice those behaviors, they won't develop diabetes. Remember, it is a predisposition, not a predetermination.

"I got it," Mary responded. "It's like a purebred horse. It could be a very well-trained horse if people work at it. But if the horse is not trained, it won't realize its potential."

"Yes, very similar," I said. "Now let me answer the other part of the question. There is a part of your physique that you cannot manipulate because you have a body type that can't change. There are three body types: ectomorph, mesomorph, and endomorph. An ectomorph is a typical skinny person with a small frame and bone structure. Ectomorphs have small joints and bones, long arms and legs, small shoulders, small muscles, small chest, and small buttocks. The ectomorph has a low body fat percentage. He or she finds it difficult to gain weight. The endomorph body type is round with medium or large joints and bones, short extremities, high levels of body fat, and a pear-shaped body. Having big undeveloped muscles makes it harder for the endomorph to lose weight. The mesomorph is naturally muscular with medium-size joints and bones with shoulders that are wider than the hips—the chest dominates over the abdominal area. The mesomorph can gain muscle quickly, but they can't lose fat easily. These body types are not written in stone, though. Most people have a combination of two body types. These combinations are either ectomorph/mesomorph or mesomorph/endomorph."

Mary was listening intently, and although I paused in case she had any questions, she let me continue.

"Many people compare themselves with other body types," I explained. For example, some ectomorphs want to have the curvy hips and chest that the endomorph has. Some endomorphs want to be thin like the ectomorph. Here is where people need to accept their bodies and make the most out of themselves. It's one thing to be overweight or have an unhealthy lifestyle, and it's another to obsess about the way one looks. Achieve a healthy weight, get the best from your body, accept your body type, don't compare yourself with others, and be happy. Simple, right?"

Mary and I smiled. We had been talking for so long that we had forgotten about the time. She was enjoying learning, and I was enjoying teaching her. But she needed to continue her day, and I needed to continue with my goals.

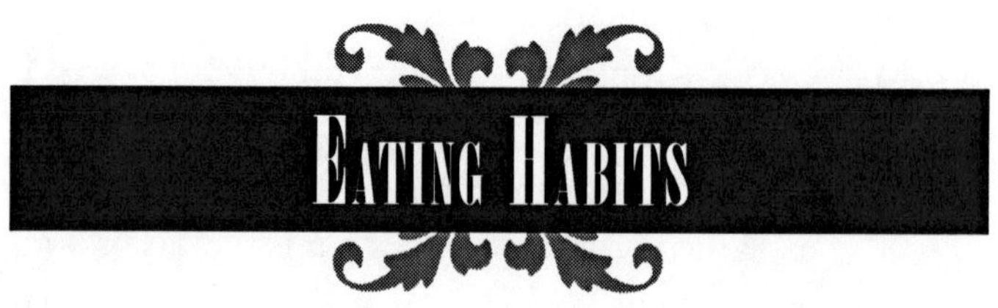

Eating Habits

Julie wanted to know more about changing her eating habits, so she called me to make an appointment about an hour after Mary left the studio. We agreed to meet the next day before the session started.

Julie said she was very confused about the information she was gathering from the Internet, nutritionists, doctors, and others. It's not surprising that she found conflicting information. I told her I'd tell her what I know and do my best not to confuse her more. So I started explaining it to Julie.

"The author Michael Pollan's research led to a simple conclusion: Eat veggies, fruits and grains; follow a low-meat diet; don't eat too much; and stay away from ultra-processed foods. In other words, do not adopt the Western diet. In his book *Unlimited Power*, Anthony Robbins also talks about confusing information on foods in American society. Back when he was ready to lose weight, he claims to have read books from authors with MDs who could not even agree on the basics. They would contradict themselves with diets and myths. Robbins says he was not looking for credentials. What he wanted was results. He shares his success of weight loss by following just six simple rules. Just like Pollan, Robbins tells us to stick to the basics."

Julie said that she needed to know more about eating and to stop being confused about food and following the masses.

The next day, Julie was on time for our meeting. I invited her to my office.

"It's good to see you, Julie," I said, starting the conversation.

"It's good to see you, too," she replied.

"How can I help you?"

"I don't know where to start," she answered, "but I'll just talk, and I hope I can help myself understand. I have being dieting for a while now. My mom used to tell me that I was fat, and I needed to do something to lose weight. There are other things that affected me, too. But what my mom told me—and my perception of my body—made me feel fat. I felt discriminated against. Many people don't understand how difficult is to have some extra pounds, not only physically but psychosocially. People don't treat us like humans. They judge us. There is more behind my story. But this is one of the reasons why I started dieting. Weight loss is the topic everywhere, and dieting is come along with it. Because everyone diets, I started dieting when I was around thirteen. Dieting has become part of my life. It is frustrating, because I don't see an end to it. Every time I go to a doctor or nutritionist, they put me on a diet. So I had thought dieting was normal until you told me the contrary."

Julie was talking from her heart and letting everything come out. I knew she needed to be heard. I have accumulated a lot of knowledge over the years, because I do a lot of research. But I'm also human, and I have been in difficult situations myself. I have felt depressed, hurt, powerless, and manipulated. Therefore, I do my best to empathize with my clients. I listen to more than their words. Sometimes it's just difficult to understand what someone's feelings and struggles are unless we've suffered the same.

Julie continued. "I really don't want to diet," she said, "and it's affecting my psychological and physical health, as you said, but I don't know what to do. I feel like I'm trapped with dieting every time I go to a professional."

"Thank you for sharing," I said. "I understand what you mean. I also see it everywhere. This is the reason why I don't recommend diets. I understand what you mean about dieting. And I'm glad you came and talked to me about it. I know there are details in your life that you may not want to share about dieting. And I know it's not an easy pattern to break. Nevertheless, here is what I can tell you about why many people prescribe or recommend diets. I once was very confused. And I discovered that the world is full of people who are not genuine. They work only for the money, and they believe what others say without thinking for themselves. They study theories they don't even understand. They live life only for living. On the other hand, you will find people who care about you, who are very ethical, and who care about your problem enough to help you. The reason I'm telling you this is because you are going to find three types of professionals: those who work for the money, those who follow theories without using common sense, and those who work for the people. Those who work for the money usually are lazy and don't do real research, even though they have a credential. They follow a textbook, believing that what they read is true. They don't understand what they are recommending. They don't even follow their own advice. Those who just believe what the population believes just believe in myth, and usually their information is not accurate. Those who care about you have committed to finding an answer for your problems, and they usually have experienced a problem like you and they have overcome the problem. These professionals read testimonials by other successful people. They don't just learn theories; they understand them. If there is a contradiction about any subject, they make sure they give you enough information to help you understand before you make a decision. And they practice what they preach. An example of a professional who cares about you is someone who will not only recommend a treatment, pill, or supplement for you to take. This professional will give you the reasons why you should take the treatment, pill, or supplement. He or she will give you other options if there are other options—which there usually are. Also, the professional will tell you all the side effects of the treatment, pill, or supplement that you are about to start. He or she is aware of any harm it can do to your health. This includes diets."

As a professional, it is hard to refer my clients to any other professional. My network is small, but I make sure all in my network are in that third category of professionals—the ones who care. I continued sharing my insight with Julie.

"What I can tell you is that I needed a lot of help when I was in depression. I found a book that answered many of my questions. Since then, I understand that I need to continue learning and that there are wiser people in the world who I need to learn from. I read all types of books: testimonials, biographies, self-help, real-life novels, and textbooks. I also go to seminars and workshops, listen to audiotapes, and find knowledgeable friends. When I go to any professional for help, I ask myself some questions: Is this person treating me like a person or a patient? Do I like him or her? Is this person listening to my concerns or does he want to tell me what he tells everyone? I recommend that you ask yourself these same questions. I'm limited. I can help you to answer many of your questions. But there is nothing like doing your own research, gathering input from other ethical people, and then coming to your own conclusions."

"I feel like you care about me," Julie said as she smiled. "What can you tell me about changing my eating habits? I was thinking yesterday after I left that I really want to change."

I reached for my notebook in my backpack. I started to write down the list of foods that contribute to unhealthy behaviors. She looked attentively at the list as I was writing it.

High fructose corn syrup: a factor in obesity (Lin et al., 2012)

- *You'll find this product in most industrialized foods.*

Processed food and genetically modified organisms: a factor in cancer, allergies, gastrointestinal and autism disorders (Conspirafied0, 2012). *They also contribute to obesity* (Canella et al., 2014).

- *Processed foods are formulated predominantly or entirely from industrial ingredients and typically contain little or no whole foods. They often have preservatives and cosmetic and other additives and may also contain synthetic vitamins and added minerals. Examples include cake mixes, energy bars,*

> *instant packaged soups, and noodles; many types of sweetened breads, cakes, biscuits, pastries, and desserts; potato or corn chips and other types of sweet, fatty, or salty snack products; sugared milk and fruit drinks, soft drinks and energy drinks; preprepared meats, fish, vegetable, or cheese dishes; pizza and pasta dishes, burgers, French fries, poultry, and fish nuggets or sticks; bread and other cereal products; sausage, hot dogs, and other products made with scraps or remnants of meat; preserved chocolates, cookies, biscuits, candies; and margarines. Also included are canned or dehydrated soups and infant formulas, and baby products.*

Industrialized meat: a factor in cancerous tumors, cancer, and sexual dysfunction (Osborne, 2011). *It also contributes to obesity* (Tunick, 2005).

- *Usually these meats have been raised with hormones and antibiotics and fed foods that the animal is not designed to eat.*

Julie had a question mark on her face when I handed out the sheet, so I started to explain.

"You can probably eat almost any food on earth," I said. "They won't affect your health negatively and you would start losing weight if you eat them with moderation. But the products on this sheet are not foods. They are called foods because humans and some domestic animals eat them. But the reality is that these products should not be eaten. This is one reason people are overweight and have so many diseases.

I learned that the human body adapts to any source of food, except the Western, fast-food diet. This is because we eat a lot of meat and processed foods that often include hormones, preservatives, chemicals, and added refined sugars and salts. Humans are designed to eat food, not chemicals; no wonder the body develops so many diseases in reaction to these processed products we eat. According to Michael Pollan, a study was conducted that introduced the Western diet to primitive hunters who normally killed and cooked their own food. These people developed medical problems just like ours: high blood sugar levels, low insulin levels, high cholesterol, high blood pressure, and others. Happily, two weeks after they went back to their native habitat and food sources, these problems disappeared.

Clearly, there is something wrong with the Western diet. This is the reason that I never encourage diets. You should not be stopping yourself from eating any real food that you want. The only guidelines are to eat natural, organic food that are not processed or treated by chemicals or other harmful products. Processed products were not made to be eaten; they were made for profit. Also, keep in mind that you should not be overeating. You want to lose weight and stay healthy? Avoid any processed food, including fast food. Let me add also that if you think that by eating vegetables you are safe, think again. Yes, vegetables are generally safe, but only if they are grown without pesticide."

"What do you mean?" she asked.

"Chemically-based pesticides make vegetables become harmful. Let me tell you about some research I did." I paused for a couple of seconds to put my ideas in order and remember my trip back to Mexico in 2013.

"When I came back from my wonderful and eye-opening vacation to Mexico City and Chiapas, I had learned more and reinforced much of my knowledge. Back in 2010, my brother was interested in having a unique pet, an iguana. When we adopted it, we had many questions, so we asked the clerk at the pet store and searched online for information about how to care for an iguana. We found out that we could feed it only organic plants. If we were to feed it other 'regular' plants, it would die. After that discovery I asked myself a deep question. Why can't the iguana eat 'regular' greens sold in the supermarket but we can? Iguanas have a lifespan of twenty years. Humans have a lifespan of 100 to 115 years. The iguana dies faster with regular foods because it develops cancer or other diseases. We have to take into consideration that the iguana lives only twenty years. Some members of my family have lived in Chiapas all their lives. For example, my grandfather is now ninety-five years of age. He walks alone, carries concrete blocks, digs holes, sweeps, and he still dresses himself. He grew up in an environment different from what many of us are living in, but this is another story. In Chiapas, it was very difficult to find someone with a chronic disease and even harder to find someone with cancer. There is a county called Emiliano Zapata in Chiapas, Mexico. There were only five hundred people. The news media brought to the public a disaster that was happing to this county. They discovered that eighty out of the five hundred people had colon cancer. And guess what? This began when the county started fumigating their natural resources with chemicals, including the mango trees, in hopes of increasing production and profit. So they were blaming this problem on the fumigation. To me it's common sense, like *one plus one is two*. Let me explain further." I was so into the conversation, and she was really into listening to me.

"According to Chiapas agriculture, a mango tree fruits three times each season. However, the first two batches of mango do not develop to an eating stage. They stay green and then go bad. The only one that reaches the eating stage is the third generation, and once it starts growing, it takes about a month to mature to an edible stage. Companies will buy all the mango batches, but farmers need to fumigate the first two stages of fruit production. By fumigating the first stage of mango production, it will take around one day to be in an edible stage. Interestingly enough, these pesticides are not safe for the people who spray them, so they need to wear special outfits that protect them from breathing the pesticides or having them come into contact with their skin. Taking that into consideration, why it is safe to eat this food contaminated with pesticides when farmers can't even breathe it or touch it? There are many studies that show how dangerous pesticides are, but people still want to save a couple of dollars by buying the 'traditional foods.' To make matters worse, companies will pay more for the mango that has been fumigated than the last batch of mango that has not been contaminated with pesticide, and that has encouraged farmers to fumigate their mango crops. My point is that besides hurting ourselves and shortening our lives by more or less 50 percent, we are supporting fumigating our food—which affects other people and the planet earth. I will ask you to be conscious about what are you are eating, which is very important to you, your family, and others. Do your best to buy products that are in season, buy locally, support the farmers that grow real food for you to eat, and buy organic. Remember, it will not do any good if you lose weight and develop a disease. Your hard work will go straight down the drain. Plus, many processed foods also contribute to the obesity epidemic. In the end, we are losing weight to be happy, and illness does not contribute to happiness is what I think."

Julie was amazed by the new information. Her eyes looked like a Japanese cartoon, big and round. Once she absorbed what I had told her, she asked, "What happened to the iguana you adopted?"

Indifferently I replied, "The iguana died."

"You fed it fumigated vegetables until it died?"

"No, the iguana died not because we didn't feed it organic, but because the heater was not hot enough in winter."

She laughed and continued talking about her habits. "Sometimes I'm running late for work, and I stop by the gas station and buy meals already made. What do you have to say about that? You recommend that people should be eating from three to five times a day, right? Is it better to eat poorly or to skip meals?"

"You should be eating three to five times a day to avoid overeating. And because you have food in your stomach, you'll be less hungry and will be more likely to choose the right foods. Hunger is a normal feeling; it's a sign that we need to eat. When we don't eat at our regular time, we can barely think because we get so hungry. In those situations, we choose foods without thinking much about them, and that will inevitably include bad products. In addition, we overeat because we continue to feel hungry after we've actually eaten enough. My clients' testimonials support this; they say that when they are hungry, they do exactly what I just told you. Plus, they get anxious, angry, and emotional. When you eat three meals and one or two snacks, you don't allow your body to get to the 'hunger' phase."

I noticed that I gave her information about her question, but I had not answered it, so I got back on track and started answering her first concern.

"Eating three to five times a day does not mean eating junk food. Many foods that you find in most gas stations is going to be junk. There may be some exceptions, but I can't come up with any. Here your problem is not giving yourself enough time to make something fast at home. If you got up ten to thirty minutes earlier, you could make yourself a smoothie, oatmeal, a bowl of fruit, a sandwich, or anything that you like to eat in the morning. What I do is give myself enough time to make a bowl of oatmeal. After I get out of bed, I go straight to the kitchen and pour the right amount of oatmeal and water into a pan and let it cook on low while I shower. When I'm out of the shower and dressed, my oatmeal is ready for me."

"The packaged food that I buy in the gas station is not good for me?" Julie asked. "Why? I don't want to get up ten minutes earlier."

"Foods that are sold in the gas station most likely are going to be industrialized food or processed foods. This is why I gave you the list of products that you should avoid," I explained.

"Oh, I see. These products can be found everywhere, not only at the supermarket. Is it the same deal with fast foods?"

"Yes, it is. Fast food chains are corporations, and they buy cheap products to make a profit. However, there are some fast foods restaurants that are aware of this problem, and they do their best to buy organic and to avoid GMOs and ultra processed foods. But these restaurants will specify that their foods are safe. Don't lie to yourself and believe that fast-food restaurant chains will have real food. If you don't want to get up ten minutes before your regular time, then you have a bad habit of eating an unhealthy breakfast. It is always up to you. You decide if you want to change your bad habit and defeat the problem that you've been trying to defeat for years. And if you think you're just making a temporary change, you may end up regaining the weight that you lose."

"I think it's worth it to get up ten minutes earlier to get rid of this extra fat I'm carrying," Julie said.

"Okay," I said and took the opportunity to talk about the next eating habit. "Cooking is one of the most important behaviors to help you lose weight and stay healthy. Michael Pollan also emphasizes this behavior. He said that by cooking you can know what are you cooking and where your foods come from. He also explains that corporations cook much differently than families do. They use lots of fat, salt, and sugar because these products are addicting. These corporations also used high fructose corn syrup. In addition, he mentions a study in which families who cook, even if they are poor, are healthier than families who don't cook. The habit of cooking contributes significantly to our health and weight loss. So you should take into consideration cooking almost all your meals at home.

This also leads me to the next recommendation: time management. One of my clients said that she is busy and doesn't have time to cook. I'm only concluding that you are in the same situation.

"Yes, I'm always running. How did you know?" she responded.

"Because many people share behaviors in their society. I make mistakes once in a while guessing since, of course, not everyone is the same. But that makes me think … do you have time to watch TV?"

Julie thought about her answer and finally said, "Yes, I do, but that is the only free time that I have to deal with my stress. Don't tell me, you guessed because many people practice this behavior as well?" she asked.

I smiled and continued. "Watching television is not a way to deal with stress, but we are going to talk about that later. Let's focus on time management. Here, let me tell you a story: The other day I had a conversation with someone who was interested in starting an exercise program. Let's call her Penelope. She has many things to do, with two sons, a husband, and work. In fact she would admit to you that she has a very stressful life. However, I have other clients who are in the same boat, yet they make the extra effort that it requires to get the healthy body they want and be happy."

I had Julie's attention, so I continued my story.

"Penelope told me that her sons are first in her life and that she doesn't really want to take time away from them to exercise. She said this even though she admits that she is not happy being overweight. Of course, I didn't counsel her to forsake her loved ones. But it seems to me that often people waste more time surfing on the web, watching television, or doing other unproductive activities—instead of investing time in something that will benefit both their bodies and their minds. Talking with Penelope reminded me of a conversation I had with a young man recently. He was confused about life and had some problems. He confided to me that he felt alone and not accepted by his dad. He even started to cry as we were talking and told me something that I will never forget: 'I don't understand, the Bible says that I need to give before I can get, and people say that I need to take care of myself before I can give.'

At the time, I told him, 'I understand your confusion. The truth is that both are right. You just need to understand it. Before you can give, you have to have it. If you don't love yourself, you can't give love to others. If you don't have money, you can't give it to someone who needs it. If you don't feel safe, you can't make someone else feel safe. It's not that we should be selfish. Care about yourself, learn, get it, understand it, and once you are blessed, then give it and care about others.'

I told Penelope that to be able to give the best to her family, she needed to care about herself a bit more. It wouldn't do her any good if she worked like a machine, giving everything with no thought to herself. You have to take care of your health to be able to give the best to your family. And there's the other concept that a parent needs to set an example for his or her family. Sometimes in my own family, I hear an adult tell a youngster to go to college, and the adult makes excuses that he or she is too old to go back to school. But this is nothing but excuses. If you want people to do something good for themselves or to make the right decisions, be a role model and do something for yourself, so in the future you are not a burden on them. To conclude, if you really want it, you can get it. All it takes is an extra effort that, sadly, many won't make. Invest your time in something that is beneficial for you and get rid of bad habits. There are other people in the same situation or even more difficult situations who have done it. Help yourself so that you'll be able to help others."

I looked away and then back at her hoping that she understood that the problem wouldn't be solved if she didn't see the importance of time management—and that she had some negative habits that she did not want to give up, such as watching television.

"The only way you can start cooking, losing weight, and maintaining your health is by making time for the new good habit—in this case cooking. Plan your day and think about all your priorities, including your health and your family. If you put cooking before television, you'll find that you'll start losing weight, you'll feel better, you'll have some quality time with your family, and cooking will help you with your stress, guaranteed."

Julie finally understood that she was making excuses because she did not want to cook. There is something inside of us that makes it difficult to start a good habit. But once we get the momentum going, it gets easier. This could explain why many people see obstacles in their journey and they become excuses. However, as the go alone with the program, those excuses diminish.

"Okay, I will start planning my day and make cooking a priority," she said.

I wanted Julie to understand the importance of her habits, so I re-emphasized, "If you don't plan your day and make good habits a priority, you will pay the consequences—some of which you are already dealing with. You hired me to help you achieve your goals. And I will. My job is to help you see the reality of your life, but you need to make the effort."

"I got it, I will do it," she said. "You told me before that the problem was not my body but the lifestyle I'm leading. So I guess I need to change some of my habits, and cooking is one of them. I really want to lose weight and feel better. I will do what it takes, and I know you are telling me all this because you want me to succeed in my weight loss goal."

I was happy she understood my point and that she decided to change some of her habits. I knew I had provided her with a lot of information, so I summarized it on a single piece of paper where I also listed the foods to avoid. "Here," I said, "This is an example of my day. This does not mean that you need to eat the same. Find what you like, and just follow the guidelines that we have been discussing since you started the program."

> *4:30 a.m.: A bowl of oatmeal with raisins and water, cooked on the stove*
> *10 a.m.: 1/3 of kefir yogurt with an apple*
> *1–2 p.m.: Scrambled organic egg with broccoli, bell peppers, tomatoes, and onions and with organic double fiber bread*
> *4–5 p.m.: Fruit (apple, banana, pear)*
> *8–9 p.m.: Anything cooked (chicken stew with vegetables and rice)*

> *My lunch and dinner usually consist of 60 to 70 percent vegetables, 20 to 30 percent grains, and 10 to 20 percent protein coming from meat.*

"Eat more vegetables and fruits than anything else. And I'll also write the rules that I follow," I said as I continued writing.

1. *Eat 3 to 5 times a day*
2. *Eat breakfast within 30 minutes of when you wake up*
3. *Stay away from ultra processed foods*
4. *Cook at home*
5. *Eat fruits and vegetables in high percentage*
6. *Cut down your meat intake*
7. *Eat organic*
8. *Drink only water*

Julie glanced at the paper and said that drinking solely water would be difficult for her. I compared the behavior of eating healthy with marriage: "Changing your eating habits is like a marriage; if you want the benefits, you must take the whole package."

She responded, "Marriage is not easy."

I replied, "You're right. I never said changing habits is easy. Anything in life that is worthwhile requires responsibility, commitment, dedication, and discipline."

"Do you eat carbs?" she asked.

"Yes, I eat brown rice, whole wheat organic pasta and anything that is not refined, processed with chemicals, or harmful to my health. It must be organic. Good carbohydrates are not the problem, because they actually contribute positively to your health. They fuel the nervous system, are used for intense and fast movements and contain fiber, which helps you lose weight among other benefits. Bad carbohydrates include refined pastas, sugar, bread, processed pastries, and other ultra processed foods that negatively contribute to your health and promote obesity. It's okay to eat a pastry once in a while, but make sure it's homemade or fresh and made locally. I eat pastries maybe every three weeks. There is nothing wrong with eating pastries in moderation and made with good ingredients.

Julie was contemplating the sheet like someone who just found an old book that she knew had good information, but she was not interested in reading it back in the past. Now Julie was ready to absorb the information. I could see hope in her eyes. Then, I concluded the conversation.

"There always will be consequences no matter what habits you are practicing. This is what you need to know: There always will be consequences. The truth is that if you continue practicing the same habits over and over again, you will have a predictable result. Negative habits will always bring negative results, and good habits will bring you success. Albert Einstein said, 'Insanity is doing the same thing over and over again and expecting different results.' Think about this," I said with a wink. "Changing your eating habits is the key to success. It is not about restricting foods but about learning the real consequences of the food you're eating and learning about processed food. Cook at home, and don't eat as a convenience at a fast food restaurant. Eat each of your three meals and your snacks; skipping meals will lead you to overeat or eat the wrong foods. Buy real food, buy organic, avoid hormones and pesticides that contribute negatively to your health, plan your day, and don't let hunger catch you off guard. Usually you will eat whatever's easiest when you're very hungry. Learn about what foods your body likes. And overall, enjoy your food, and don't be at war with the products that make you healthy. I believe in you," I said with a smile.

Many people are very excited when they gather new information, and they are ready to apply it right away. Many people change for short period of time, sometimes weeks or months, but then they go back to their old habits. I always hope that people understand that they need to change their habits forever. They need to continually learn and apply new information in their lives. When I have any conversation about habits, it reminds me of when one of my clients approached me and told me that since she overeats cookies, she was giving up cookies for Lent and that forty days later she would go back to the same habit. I thought about how much good forty days would be in helping her achieve her goal. I concluded that it was a waste of time for her to give up cookies for only forty days. She needed to understand that giving up cookies for forty days wouldn't help her achieve her long-term goal. She needed to change her perception about cookies. She needed to change her eating behavior forever, not for just forty days. Thanks to her, I realized I had made some mistakes in my life. I remember wanting to give up a negative behavior for only thirty days. When she made the comment about *giving up cookies for Lent* I caught myself having done the same. So at the time I understood that if I wanted positive results in my life, I needed to change my negative behaviors forever, not for thirty or forty days.

Perception to Reality

Julie, Mary, and the other members were ready to start the training session. I begin with a short speech. We all need some words of encouragement to help us reach our goals. Some of us think that everyone knows what we know or that everyone thinks and sees the world as we do. When we think that, we make a big mistake. Many people don't see, feel, or perceive the world as we do. If we take it for granted that someone knows something and we leave it at that, we probably won't make the impact we want to make. It is important to express and deliver the message effetely, so people do understand and see things as we want them to see them. Here is my speech:

"In life we find people who succeed in their goals and others who will only try. To be more specific, less than 8 percent of people will succeed in their weight-loss goals. There are people who have every reason to succeed in their weight-loss goals but still fail. Then there are others that have less chance to achieve their goals yet succeed. What is the difference between these two types of people? The consequences obviously are not a factor. Sidike Conde is a great example; with no legs he could achieve more than people with legs. The way people perceive life is the biggest factor in why people succeed or fail. I was talking to my

landlord the other day, and she was telling me how some tenants are full of excuses. Even though they have every chance to stay on top of things, they prefer to leave everything to the last minute and then come up with all types of excuses. Interestingly enough we are all full of excuses. We blame anyone and/or everything, but we don't take responsibility for our own life decisions.

Here, I'll illustrate using two different people, same event: One is doing her best to lift weights and get out of her comfort zone. Every time she is squatting she thinks, 'The burn and the pain will help me lose fat and get my legs and butt toned. I can do this: no problem. I have done it before. I like this feeling of accomplishment.' When she is running, she tells herself, 'Running is only for the strong, and I'm strong. I can run twenty miles. My body was made to run.' When she chooses to eat the right foods, her inner thoughts are, 'My life is healthier with these foods. Healthy foods are the best energy I can consume for my body.' The second person, when she is squatting, says, 'Oh no, this is very difficult. My legs are killing me. I can't do this. I will never get what I want. I should stop now.' She comments to herself while running, 'It seems too long. My body can't handle the running. I'd better walk, because running does not feel comfortable.' When she chooses what to eat she says, 'I will only eat processed foods once. Why should I cook when there is food that is already made? Processed foods are the easiest thing to eat, and I don't care about my health anyway, because I will still die someday."

Can you feel the joy of one of them and the pain of the other? If you picture these two people, I would hope that you would want to be the first. I could be wrong. Maybe you would want to be example number two and continue making excuses. I know you are smarter than that. Anyway, did you notice that both these people in the same event were affected differently by how they perceived the same event? The reality is that you create your reality. You are the one who decides if it is painful or enjoyable. How do you perceive events?"

My speech was over, and all my clients where ready to exercise. I perceived that I delivered the message, and they were ready to do what it takes to get to their goals.

After an hour of exercise, everyone was happy that it was over. One of the members asked me why I love to exercise and how I found passion in it. I replied to him that exercise is not what gets me going; the feeling of lifting weights, lacking oxygen, or burning muscles is not what I look for. What makes me passionate about lifting weights, increasing my heart rate and feeling the burn is the result that exercise gives me. Also, the feeling of accomplishing my goal of the day, the feeling of giving every effort I could give when I exercise. My client liked the way I think. After the session, she asked me for another example of how to perceive events, so I told her the following analogy:

"I read about a teacher in a third-world country where the school was built with very cheap materials. It could barely stand up, and the rain and wind would cause major damage to the buildings. One day a storm came and took all the buildings as if they were pieces of paper. The children in the town had nowhere to study. The teacher said that it was a great opportunity for her. She found the way to open a nonprofit through which many people found out about the situation. So people sent contributions, and the teacher saved more than enough money to build the school with better materials. When the school was finished, it was a place where children were proud to go study. Was the storm devastating? The reality is how people perceive it. From the standpoint of a negative person, it would have been a disaster and the end of her career and her dream. For this teacher it was the beginning of a new opportunity, and it was one of the best things that could have happened to her. Once again, same event, different perceptions; both realities are true, but which one would you choose? All you have to do is pay the price and get out of the comfort zone. And this is true for all your thoughts."

"So, if we see the world with positive perception, there really isn't anything bad, right?" she asked.

"No, everything that happens is for your own benefit and for your personal growth. Tragedies help many people to get out of their comfort zone. This is the reason why many nonprofit organizations exist. I was told about an organization where many leaders from Latin America get together to collect the resources to help with blood and bone marrow transfusions for people with leukemia. They connect those in need with donors. And they will raise money to pay for the expenses. The reason why these leaders get together is because they all have something in common; they lost a loved one to leukemia. I personally think that there's a message, a wake-up call, or a reminder about our power and purpose when we experience tragedies."

"However," she said, "there are people who will be destroyed by pain. This is due to their perception of the event, as you were saying."

"Yes, keep in mind that I'm not saying the event is pain-free. Also, the willingness to pay the price to overcome the pain is a big factor that many are not willing to pay."

"So I should suffer when I exercise to be able to achieve my goals?" She smiled sarcastically and in a playful manner.

"No. Suffering is a perception. However, you don't want to put yourself in a situation where pain is not fun anymore. Many people don't have to lose a loved one to understand their purpose and open a nonprofit to help others. Getting out of your comfort zone requires effort and discomfort but not pain. Exercising gives you a burn, fatigue, and soreness, but not pain. Many people call those feelings pain, but they're not."

"Oh," she responded. "I need to be more aware about what I'm feeling when I exercise and not tell my brain that it's pain if it's a burn, fatigue, or soreness. I can perceive it with a positive attitude."

"You hit the target. Now keep in mind that you need to practice your perception, and soon it will become automatic."

Every night I do a summary of my day in my head. I usually sit on my bed to think. According to Henry Ford, *Thinking is the hardest work there is, which is probably the reason why so few engage in it.* Even though I agree with Henry, I think it's like any other habit. It becomes easier as you continue practicing. I thought about the conversation that I had with my clients that day. Sometimes when people get divorced or a relative dies, they expose their pain to others. They like the attention that others give them. Usually, they use their pain as an excuse not to live their reality. One of my clients also went through the same thing, and she told me she could talk to me because we are like rehabbed alcoholics; we could understand each other's pain. I laughed when she told me that, but it's true. Many people don't understand the situation. I used the pain to succeed and got rid of the demons that kept me chained to my bad habits. In contrast, I have met many people that get lost in alcohol, drugs, or other bad habits for the same reason. This is also applicable to overeating and other bad habits that contribute to being overweight. I thought about the many people who are covering depression with these bad habits, and they don't want to confront the pain. I could not stop thinking about events. When a painful event occurs, many people want to cover the pain with bad behaviors because of the prompt gratification they can provide. But it's clear that thoughts are what create the pain. And many people try to repress their painful thoughts. And this is like hiding a dead animal in a closet; sooner or later it will stink and bring parasites to the house. So the best solution is to deal with those painful thoughts. But how? So I concluded that those thoughts are what people usually call stress. The body releases hormones accordantly to our thoughts. We can be on *fight or flight* with our thoughts and the body will release the hormones require accordantly to the action it thinks it will take.

I got out of bed, got my notebook and a pen, and I started to undo the riddle by writing down all the information that was collected in my head.

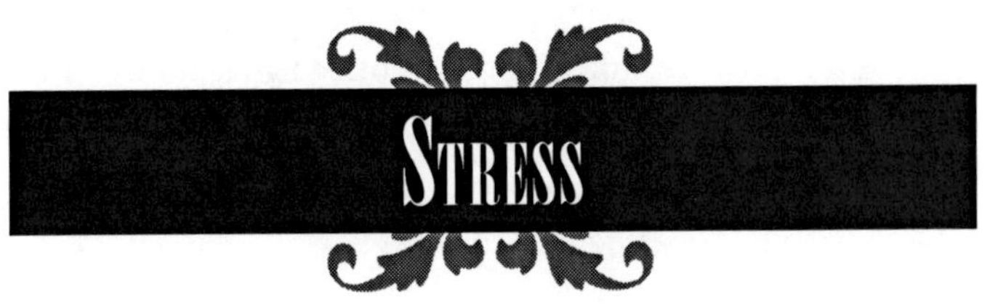

Stress

I know that stress is one of the most problematic conditions in the world. It has been linked to diseases such as cancer, sleep disorders, eating disorders, weight problems (obesity and anorexia), heart diseases, hypertension, depression, schizophrenia, drug addiction, alcoholism, immune system weakness, and others. Many people recommend superficial ways to deal with stress such as massages, and going on vacation. These things do help us relax, but relaxing doesn't really help us understand what we're dealing with. Stress is caused by thoughts that trouble us, problems that we need to solve, or questions we need an answer to. Dealing with different problems requires different levels of mental energy. For example, a divorce takes a lot of energy thinking about the time invested in the marriage, the plans to do things together, how children will react, learning to live single, making decisions alone, economic changes, and so on. A broken-down car is less stressful; depending on the person's situation, he or she can fix it, buy another one, or take it to the junkyard. The two events may both be stressful, but the reality is that a divorce requires a lot more energy. There are emotions, time, family, plans, dreams, memories, and friends involved. In comparison, a car is a tool that we use to transport ourselves from point A to point B.

I was writing and making sense. Writing is important for me because I can record my thoughts and go back at any time to review my conclusions. I noticed that many of my ideas come from reading the research and studies of other authors, but I understand the idea and put it in my own words with my own perspective.

Past Stress

As I continued writing, I thought about how people don't live in the moment. Many people are stuck in the past, thinking about what could have been, what they no longer have, or what they once accomplished. I've heard some people say things like: "If I had the job I had before, I'd be happy"; "If I hadn't lost the money in stocks, I could buy myself that house"; or "If I had only stayed in school, I would have a degree." People stress out about the past. They don't think about the resources they have now. They don't understand that what's important is what they have now and what they can do now. People who live in the past often can't forgive themselves or others. Therefore, they are stressed most of the time. They waste a lot of energy. A massage won't release the stress permanently, nor will an exercise class. Vacation won't do it, either. These things can help people relax mentally and give them the opportunity to deal with their stress, but if they keep thinking about their past, the stress will continue. Sometimes these thoughts lead to anger, bitterness, or other negative feelings.

It was a full moon. I could see the moon from my window, and I could hear the crickets sing. Otherwise, the bright night was quiet. Conditions were perfect for me to keep thinking. My brain works better when there are no manmade distractions. Because I was concluding that people stress about the past, I decided to call it *past stress*, where people continue to drag their past into the present. I remember when I asked a friend about a relationship that didn't turn out the way she would have liked. I believe her boyfriend cheated on her. She told me she didn't remember much about that guy and that it was a long time ago. But when she told me about it, I could detect some bitter feelings. Sometimes people try to repress uncomfortable thoughts, and they try to forget. The reality is that the mind can't forget stressful events. The way to deal with past stress is to confront the situation, understand why it happened, forgive, and move forward with one's life. This can be compared to posttraumatic stress disorder. Most people who have been through an extremely traumatic event cannot forget easily, and they are emotionally scarred forever. To cope with PTSD, some people turn to recreational, legal, or prescription drugs, which can lead to substance abuse and addiction.

It was getting late. I needed to wake up early in the morning, but I was so into writing that I didn't care about the time. I don't write every night, and the ideas would give me insomnia anyway. The best action to take was to keep writing.

Present Stress

Trying to decide whether to write or sleep made me think about "present stress." What type of things do people get stressed about in the present? I came up with money, work, bills, and vacation. But do people really need to stress out about all these things? This question led me to consider two types of present stress: stressing about something that contributes positively to our lives and that which contributes negatively to our lives. The reality is that stress that contributes positively to our life can contribute negatively to it as well, depending in how we perceive the stress. I used a car payment as an example. For some people a car is a necessity. It is hard to find reliable transportation in some areas of the world. A car is needed to save time, be more efficient, and make life easier to some extent. If we buy a car within our budget or even cheaper, chances are that we'll end up paying for the car without stressing out, and if we maintain it, it may last us for quite a while. I have a car that is eleven years old that works perfectly and is in great condition. I have no stress from making payments that I can't afford. So paying for the car was stressing about something good because it was an investment. It takes me from work and back to my house, and I use it for personal trips as well. But paying for a car becomes negative stress when people opt to buy one that is not within their budget, possibly because of their self-image; they try to impress people with the car they've bought. They want to be accepted, and they feel that a car will project a better image. Of course, a salesman will make the payments sound easy and affordable. The buyer will also rationalize his decision to buy the car, not taking into consideration that maybe his family is living day-to-day and that someday he could lose that job or earn less money. Many people live day-to-day, and they can't afford what they think they can. Many people have lost their houses or cars, they're in debt with many credit cards, and they continue to make the mistake of buying things they can't afford.

I took a break but kept thinking about what else contributes to present stress, so I continued writing.

My brother and I have adopted two dogs that we love. They require food, exercise, veterinary services, training, patience, and love. They cause stress, present stress. There is never a day that I don't think about walking them. Since I care about these two members of my family, I cook organic food for them. When they need medical attention, I take them to the veterinarian. The stress they cause me is repaid by the company they give us. I love when I come home and they are waiting for me. As soon as they see me, they start wagging their tails, jumping around, barking and running from one side of the house to the other. They give me joy. In addition, thanks to adopting them, I have developed the habit of hiking or walking every day, which contributes positively to my physical and mental health. Is the stress worth it for the company they give me? In my case, it is. So these animals contribute to my life positively.

Finally, I needed to make my thoughts clearer, so I decided to summarize them.

Negative present stress is caused by things, events, or people who take energy from us, don't contribute positively to our lives, and take our hard work away from us without giving us anything in return. Positive present stress is caused by things, events, or people that contribute positively to our lives; they are useful and give us a service or value back.

A couple of hours had passed, and I was feeling a little tired, but I didn't want to go to sleep until I got all my thoughts clear in my head. Nevertheless, I changed into my pajamas, said my prayer, and went to bed, setting the alarm for early in the morning. I'm accustomed to making my body and brain tired. This way, I get to sleep and rest with no problem, just like a newborn baby. It felt like I had just touched the pillow when my alarm went off. I went straight to the kitchen, put my oatmeal in a pan, covered it with water, and put the heat on low. I showered, dressed, put some raisins in my oatmeal, sat by the table, turned my computer on, started eating, and picked up my thoughts where I left them.

Future stress

In this category people worry about things that haven't happened yet. They're afraid of getting a disease, losing their house, having an accident, getting divorced, losing their job, and so on. The problem with stress is that people put a lot of energy into their worries, affecting their lives in many ways, even causing mental and physical diseases. I have read that 75 percent of physical diseases are caused by stress. Since we are the architects of our lives, we have the ability to prevent catastrophes. Many of the diseases we have are due to the lifestyle we lead. Therefore, instead of worrying, we should start acting to change negative behaviors that may lead to disease. Learning about all types of disease will help us make better decisions about our health. On the financial side, we can make better decisions, like investing our money instead of spending it. Investing money, time and energy in one's health, mind, profession, family, spiritual development, and in material products that add value to one's life and that can be afford, are examples.

I noticed that if we plan our lives, many of our worries about the future are taken care of in the present. There is something about humans that when we know we are doing the right thing, our brain rests and doesn't stress about tomorrow. These habits have helped me be on top of my future.

I needed to write about two more things in my life that keep me from worrying about the future.

Living in the moment keeps me busy. What is going on right now is my life, my reality. When it's time to train my clients, I train them without thinking about what I did yesterday or what I need to do tomorrow. When I need to pay my mortgage, I concentrate on paying it now, not the mortgage I would have tomorrow or the house I lost yesterday. When I'm facing a friend or family member, I tell them how much I love them. I don't think about the friend or family member who died last year or the newborn who is coming. The moment is the only thing we have that is true. The past and future are not reality. Only people who live in the moment are happy and don't have negative stress in their life. Usually these individuals are thankful to have another moment. They have found a Superior Power that leads them to be in peace, which is the other thing I have found that helps me handle stress. God is a power that the human mind finds difficult to understand. It is the creator of the universe. It's a purpose for us, and when we find its way, our life goes in the right direction. We suffer when we want to succeed but live without its guidance. When we are on the right path, we know it, just as we know when we are off of it, which is one of the reasons why we worry so much about past and future. Finding God's way and putting all our trust in it is the way to deal with stress.

It was time to go. I had to be at the training studio in fifteen minutes, and I had a twenty-minute drive. I washed my dishes and put my computer in my backpack.

When I got to the studio, Erick was ready to teach the session. Everything was set to begin. Erick is my brother and my coworker. I have the good fortune to work with a valuable member of my family. Five people showed up for the session. Erick was full of energy, and he started leading the session. I watched how much my brother has grown since he started working for me. Some of our clients' comments crossed my mind: *Erick is very sweet. He pushes us more than you. You did a good job training him. Erick feels more confident now.*

Julie entered the front door. She was fifteen minutes late for the session.

"Good evening," I said, welcoming her. It was 5:45 a.m. Our session started at 5:30 a.m. Sometimes I like to make jokes so people smile.

"Good morning," she said, sounding exhausted.

"Do you want to join this group, or are you going to wait for the next one?" I asked

"I actually want to talk to you," she said.

"You came at a good time. Erick can lead the group alone. You want to follow me to my office?"

"Yes."

We walked to my office while avoiding people lifting weights, jumping ropes, battling the ropes, and doing sit-ups or other exercises. People were energetic and motivated to work out. I was happy about the atmosphere we had created. I opened the door for Julie, and she went in and sat in a chair. I closed the door and pulled up a chair to sit in front of her.

"How can I help you?"

"I'm trying to change my habits, and it is not easy, as you mentioned. I kind of know what to eat, but I noticed that I eat all the time."

"What do you mean by 'all the time'?"

"I snack on foods that are in front of me," she answered. "They're easy to reach. And when I'm not doing anything or when I'm worried, I eat. I catch myself putting something in my mouth often."

"Why are there foods in front of you?"

"It's easy to grab candy or go to the fridge and find food like cheese," she said.

"So foods are easy to access, right?"

"Yes."

"Do you eat all your meals, breakfast, lunch, and dinner?"

"I do eat my three meals, but I don't think hunger is the reason I eat. When I'm taking care of my family I don't have time to think, so I don't eat. I think I eat to keep my mind busy."

"What makes you worry?"

"I don't know. I have no stress. My financial situation is good, I have a great husband, my family is healthy and I'm healthy. I don't think I'm worried."

"I think there is something that bothers you that you aren't able to face. To me, what you are doing sounds like *emotional eating*. You are eating to keep your mind busy, as you said. When you are engaged in an activity, your brain is occupied. But there is something that you're avoiding and you may don't want to deal with. Meditation will help you understand what worries you. You are the only person who will find what is going on in your head. Are you afraid of the future?"

"No, I usually don't care about what is coming. I know that I create my future, so I do what I can do to develop a better life today," she said.

"Here, this is what I know. Many people eat to keep their brains busy, because they're afraid of facing their thoughts. I'm not certain that this is what you're doing, but it's good to consider all the possibilities and discard them as we determine that they're not applicable to you. Joyce Meyers wrote a book called *Power Thoughts,* and she talks about her struggles in life and how thoughts were affecting her. She was heading down a destructive path. She discovered that her thoughts had a lot to do with the decisions she made. Her book is amazing. She is a very knowledgeable lady, and I was surprised by the ability she has to clearly explain her topic. Many people have developed the capacity to express themselves with their soul, and I think Meyers is among them. One of the reasons I believe she's so special and successful is how she dealt with hard times. What I found very interesting is that she discloses that she was sexually abused by her father at a young age. It wasn't easy for her, but she developed the power of forgiveness. Of course, I'm not saying this happened to you, but the statistics show that one out of three women was raped at a young age. Some also suffered physical or mental abuse. And the reason why I'm bringing this up is because it could be something kind of abuse that happened on the past that you may have blocked and you don't want to think about it."

Julie was looking down, processing what I was saying. Her eyes started to water, and she paused for at least a minute before she started talking.

"It's hard for me to talk about. I was sexually abused by my uncle."

Forgiveness

Her revelation was not surprising. I have heard this story before. The statistics say that one out of three women are sexually abused. I can only imagine how high the percentage would be if all women decided to declare their incident. I read that 75 percent of these women are raped by people they know well, such as boyfriends, friends, co-workers, classmates, bosses, and relatives. Some people picture rapists waiting in the streets for the opportunity to strike. While this happens, most rapists are guys who already know their victim. They usually fantasize and plan everything out, and many times they live nearby or in the same house.

I was deep in thought but heard Julie say, "My husband has been very supportive. He knows about the incident, and I think I have not forgotten it. Maybe that could be what is bothering me. I have suffered so much; you have no idea what I have gone through."

"Julie, I have never been raped, so I can't say that I understand your pain exactly. But I also have suffered, so I can tell you that I know suffering. Keep in mind that you are not the only human being who has gone through this pain, and, though I'm not saying that your pain is nothing, there are people who have been in deeper pain than you. Nevertheless, keep in mind that they have overcome their pain. Joyce Meyer is a great example. My pain was not as deep as yours, but it was enough for me to understand that I needed to become a better person and stop making excuses in order to continue with my life and release my potential. I want you to think that people who hurt us don't do it because they want to hurt us. They are looking for their own satisfaction. They are egocentric, and they don't think about the pain and scars they are causing us. They are slaves to their own desires, and they can't control their thoughts. I read in the book *The Monk Who Sold His Ferraru* that a healthy mind is one that controls its own thoughts, while an ill mind is one that is controlled by its thoughts. These people won't be able to change until they understand they are sick. Your job is not to condemn him. Your job is to forgive him. If you don't forgive, you are the one who will suffer the consequences. It is like you drinking the poison expecting your aggressor to die. Many people live with fear, anger, resentment, and other negative emotions as a result of being abused. However, most people who have been abused don't understand that the people who abused them are also slaves to the transgressions of others. Therefore, it is hard for the abused to forgive. They remember the incident and live with negative emotions for many years, and some die with these feelings. Some people are even angry with God for the incident. But these feelings will lead people to self-destruction as they practice negative behaviors and become addictive.

For some reason I think one of the commitments says to forgive others on the Bible. Nobody told them that forgiveness will release them from their aggressor. At one point in my life I was self-destructing; it happens to many people without their realizing it. Let me add to this that many people make mistakes and can't forgive themselves, either. If it is hard to forgive someone else, it is harder to forgive yourself.

You are the worst judge of yourself. The key to dealing with past stress is to learn how to forgive others and yourself. The best way to learn about forgiveness is by learning why people do what they do. I started studying my past, and I understand my mistakes and why I made them. Once I understood my past, I could understand others. Then I learned how to forgive my transgressors and myself.

In the biography of Dr. Bernard Nathanson is an example of a past behavior as stress. Nathanson was one of the professionals who fought for legalization of abortion. He performed more than sixty thousand abortions, which he later regretted after he found out exactly what he was doing. All the abortions that he performed became past stress. Therefore, he felt guilty and developed depression. He tried different ways to escape, such as a suicide attempt, alcoholism, antidepressants, therapy, and self-help books, but nothing worked. Later in his life, he found the solution to his problem. He learned how to forgive himself, and he started to publicly broadcast what really happens in an abortion to compensate for his transgressions.

I had a client who said she had been sexually abused by her grandfather. She had resentment and anger, and she was afraid of men. Later in her life, she discovered that her grandfather had also been raped when he was a child; therefore, he was psychologically damaged and what he did was a reaction to another's transgression. She let go her negative feelings, forgave her grandfather, and moved out of his house.

Now keep in mind that I'm saying that the transgression is an excuse for people to go hurt others, but people don't really understand. She will never forget the event, but she understands why it happened, and she is free of negative feelings. What would have happened if she had put her negative feelings into work and condemned her grandfather or killed him? Don't you think the cycle would have continued? Reporting the incident to the authorities is the best thing one can do. But from then on, one can only forgive. I recommend that you read books about forgiveness. Remember that forgiveness will change your thought patterns and will release the stress that you've been carrying for years. Also, forgiveness is not justice. God will take care of that. Forgiveness is a gift you give to the aggressor and a gift you give to yourself. Forgiveness doesn't mean living with the aggressor or allowing the aggressor to keep hurting you. Forgiveness means understanding that the aggressor is ill and you need to stay away from him with the hope that he someday will understand his problem. Maybe someday he will come and genuinely apologize.

Apologizing won't let you forgive, but it will help you understand that he is human just like you and you also make mistakes. Something that you probably know is that you're still as valuable as before, or even more so since you understand what happened. You have a great family, including your husband who supports you. You must shed the extra weight you've been carrying for years now. You will never forget, but you can remember without pain. It is possible."

Julie stopped crying. She smiled and said that she has a wonderful family, and she needed to continue losing weight. She told me that the reason she wanted to lose weight was that a doctor told her she needed to. She had a liver disorder that would require surgical intervention unless she lost some weight. We continued talking about her problem, and she concluded that the extra weight was not affecting her health. It was her bad habits and the food she was eating that damaged her liver and increased her fat levels and weight. Julie said she was ready to change her life and that she would do everything in her power to keep up good habits. All she needed from me was my support. I told her that she had my support, but she needed to be patient with herself. I saw hope in her eyes. We shared some trivial conversation about how the day had gone and she continued her day.

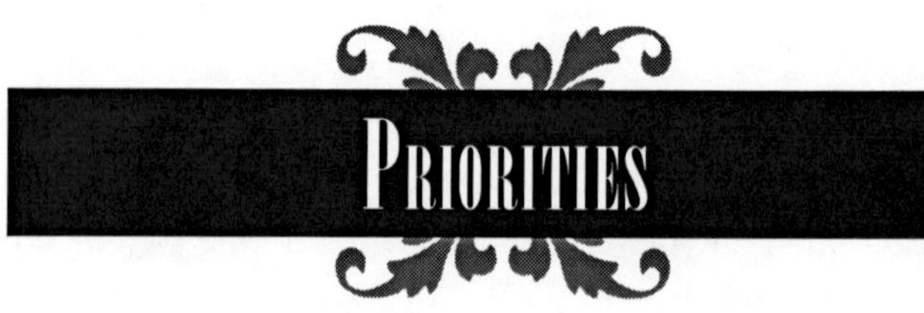

Priorities

It had been more than a month since Julie and I had our conversation about forgiveness. We were having another conversation on the phone. She said she stills weighs the same. Julie was five feet four inches tall, thirty-five years of age, weighed 219 pounds, and had 42.6 percent body fat. She said she was getting frustrated with her weight loss results because she had made some changes in her life, such as not dieting anymore. But the liver pain she had was gone, and she felt more energetic. So she was still positive about her weight-loss program despite her frustration with the scale. I told her that the weight loss would happen in time. In the meantime, we needed to go over the changes she had made to set up some specific goals so she could "touch" the changes she had made. I told her she should be happy that the liver pain was gone and that this was the real reason she had started the program. Also, I recommended that she see her doctor to make sure that there was a positive change in her liver disease.

It was the end of the day, and I gave myself some time to clear my mind. I heard in an audiotape that the brain has the ability to filter out all the things you're not interested in and absorb what you're focused on. I noticed that the conversation I had with Julie had to do with past stress, something I had been writing about the night before. I decided to send out my writing on stress in a few newsletters. One of our subscribers was interested in the content of my newsletter, especially the topic of present stress.

Hello Sandro,

Good job on your newsletter. I like the content, and I think I can put it into practice. I have a couple of questions about the topic of your newsletter: past, present, and future stress. My issue is that I get a little overwhelmed by my present stress, and I would like to know more about the subject and if you can also give me more information about future stress. Thank you.

Carmen

Hello Carmen,

Thank you for your reply, and I'm glad my emails are helpful. They are made for you to put information into practice. What type of information exactly are you looking for, so I can be more specific in answering your question?

Carmen: Sandro! I want to know what I can do to deal with my present stress. Your newsletter gives a good explanation about the stresses in life, but it doesn't explain how we can deal with it. I'm interested in knowing more about present and future stress. Can you give an explanation about how can I deal with present and future stress? Thank you.

Sandro: Yes, Carmen. Prioritizing is the best thing you can do to deal with present stress. Let me explain; present stress I think is easier to deal with. Here you need to deal with your priorities and what you want from your heart, not what others might want from you. When people do not have this concept clear, they get persuaded easily. As an example, they buy or act emotionally. Human beings need to feel accepted to be happy, and we practice behaviors that go against our beliefs or status to be accepted by our peers. This is one of the reasons why people buy things they can't afford or engage in negative behaviors like smoking or drinking. People need to consider what really contributes to their own happiness and who they want to be accepted by, so they can start prioritizing their needs and wants. For instance, people need real food to survive. If you think about the consequences of the investment in your food, you'll see that in the long run better food will keep you healthier, saving you money and pain. So one priority can be your food. Shelter is also a priority. Your physical and mental health, your family, your knowledge, your body, your spirit, and your career are priorities. You can't argue that any of these priorities are not important for your happiness. The rest are wants and needs as lower priorities. Clothing, hobbies, communication devices, traveling, eating out, movies, and television are only a few examples of lower priority wants and needs. Most people are in debt because they don't know how to separate their wants and their needs and prioritize them. Common sense says that needs are more important than wants.

In addition, there are things that need to be done every day, such as taking the kids to school, cooking, paying bills, washing dishes, studying, working, cleaning, and so on. Many people ignore some of these chores and choose to waste their time watching television or doing some other trivial thing. They know there are chores to do, but they choose to ignore them. Then later, they stress out because they don't have time to do them. My point here is if you don't want to stress out about your chores, then get them done. Just as we prioritize our needs and wants, the same thing applies to the things that have to be done. They need to be prioritized. What is more important, studying for the upcoming final or watching some random program that does not add value to your life? Which of those really will take the stress away?

I hope this explanation helps make it clear how you can approach present stress.

Carmen: You explained it well. Let me summarize. I need to determine my needs and make them top priorities of the things I need to survive, such as eating, shelter, and work. Now I can go to the next level and prioritize the things I need to progress in my life, such as a car for transportation, continuing education, and exercise. Also, I think I need to be accepted by my close loved ones, so spending time with them is a priority. Then my wants, such as vacation and luxuries like timeshares, a second car, cable television, and expensive bags and clothing that I have become obsessed about buying. What do you think? Do I have it right?

Sandro: Yes, Carmen, you understand prioritizing. Just keep in mind that you are prioritizing everything every day. Here is an example: Because your work, food, and shelter are your top priorities, you need to make the time and save the money to maintain them. You need to schedule time to clean your house, spend the right amount of money on your food, and find a job that you enjoy by getting the right training and education. Then you need to find time every day to spend with your family, husband, and children if you are married. During the day, you also need to find time to read and exercise. After you have covered every single need, then you can spend time and money on your wants. If by any chance you have time for only your needs, then your wants will be pushed to the side. Many people make the mistake of putting their needs to the side. Here is an example: They save up for a new expensive dress or watch by buying cheap food, such as fast food and ultra-processed food. Here people are prioritizing their wants instead of their needs. Let me know if all this makes sense to you.

By the way, I recommend you meditate and find all your needs and make them priorities. Some needs are obvious, like food and shelter for survival, but others are less obvious, such as studying. Many people can survive without studying, but they live their lives under the knowledge of people that are not competent to help them and this can lead people to make wrong decisions in life. Plus, people have less ability to progress in their personal life or improve their quality of life. God is my priority on top of everything. It may not sound obvious. The problem with many people is that they don't understand the concept of God. God is a verb, and God is all the positive actions. Meditation gives me a great connection with this superior power. Therefore, meditation has become a priority in my life. Just as with studying, you can survive without meditation, but that doesn't mean you're realizing your potential or improving your quality of life. Just like you have to exercise your body and mind, the spirit needs exercise as well.

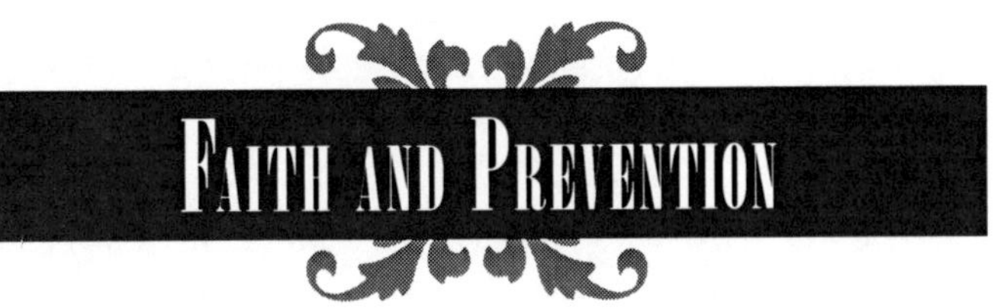

Faith and Prevention

I like taking my time explaining what I know to people. I like open-minded people who are curious and not afraid to ask questions. People like this stay young forever; they continue learning and progressing in life. They know they don't know it all. As many people grow old, they think they know it all. They become stubborn. When someone wants to share information and they've heard it before, they stop the conversation. They then lose the opportunity to refresh their memory or to hear it from a different perspective. Personally, I've learned things each time I've heard the same information repeated. When I hear it from different people, I learn it in a different way. Carmen was young but very mature and smart for her age. She replied back to remind me that I hadn't touched on how to deal with future stress.

Carmen: Everything makes sense. I have to read it over again to start prioritizing my needs and wants. I have to make sure I don't confuse my needs with my wants. Sometimes I think I need a drink to deal with stress, and I end up having two drinks and not taking care of my house. But I don't actually need to drink, so I think I can save money by not buying alcohol. I can also protect my health, because I know alcohol has many negative effects on the human body and on human behavior.

Plus, I can be cleaning my house instead of just watching my favorite reality show while having a drink.

I got it all figured out, right? Now what can you tell me about future stress?

Sandro: Carmen, you learn fast. You got it. And just for your information, you are dealing with some future stress by quitting the habit of drinking. If you continue drinking, it'll have negative consequences. You can replace this negative habit with a good one that will bring positive results in the future. Let me explain further.

People have different beliefs, and they can lead them to be afraid of some things or not to believe in themselves. Let me give you a couple of examples: A person who was kidnapped in a city might believe that cities aren't safe and be afraid that it might happen again when they're in a city. A person who has experienced cancer in her family may be afraid that she is predetermined to develop cancer. Families who have seen a friend lose their house and business can be afraid of buying a house or opening a business. These people are afraid of the unknown and have decided what their future will be like. Subconsciously, they are stressing themselves about something that isn't real and are living their lives in fear. What I do to deal with things that haven't happened yet is decide what outcome I want in the future. I learn the facts about diseases such as cancer and I void them: stress, microwaves, pesticides, hormones, plastic, aspartame, and so on. I determine my bad habits and change them to good habits that will give me positive results. For example, I learned how to manage my money and invest it in the right way, so I don't end up losing what I've fought to obtain. Someone once told me that I don't get preoccupied, I occupy myself. And what really helps me with my future stress is the ability to leave everything in God's hands. I know he has a plan for me and that I don't have control over outside sources, so I let him guide me, and I do what I can to lead my destiny in the direction I want without worrying. Outside sources over which I don't have control are the weather and other people's decisions, for example. But I do have control over how I perceive events. In addition, the lives of others are not directly dependent on me, so I enjoy my time with them, so I don't regret when they're gone. I love my brother, and I enjoy every moment with him. I love my dogs because they are part of my family. They are family members, and just like any other member I care a lot about them. Let me give you an illustration: This weekend while on a walk, my friend and I sat and started eating our lunches. My dog was a couple of feet away from me; he was acting weird, and he suddenly collapsed. I got up right away and picked him up. He wasn't responding. I ran to my car as I yelled many times telling him not to leave me now. He tried opening his eyes, but he couldn't. In my desperate attempt to save him, I stuffed my finger down his throat. I didn't know what was happening, but he could have eaten something poisonous. Green saliva came out of his mouth. He tried to react, but also could not. I didn't stop yelling or begging him not to leave. I drove to the veterinarian. The only one open was an emergency vet 25 miles away. Through the whole drive I continued to encourage my dog. He finally woke up, but with no energy. We made it to the veterinarian, and he was fine by that time. I was worried about his heart, so I had the veterinarian check his cardiac rhythm. The veterinarian tried to guess what was wrong with him, but at the same time something inside of me made me think it could've been an allergic reaction. She checked him and tried different tests. In the meantime my dog started to show hives, and we later learned it was indeed an allergic reaction. After I assimilated everything, I was happy instead of scared. I was happy because he was alive. However, if God had decided to take him, I would have been happy as well because I enjoyed every single moment with my wonderful dog. Enjoy the moment, and I'm prepared for the future by working toward the desired outcome, I leave my life in the hands of a Superior Power, and I know that everything will turn out the way it's supposed to.

By the way, I have attached a file that I read in a book called "Flying Over the Swamp."

(Attachment)

Sometimes alcohol dependence is a slow process. Everything is based on predisposition and metabolic conditions. Some people get addicted quickly, while for others it takes many years. The process, slow or fast, almost always follows the same pattern. At first, people start drinking in meetings or with friends; this first level is called a social drinker. Once people experience the misleading feeling of wellness that alcohol gives, they start drinking alone to feel relaxed and relieved of their pressures; this second level is called a relief drinker. Slowly, the body develops a defense mechanism, called tolerance, to compel the individual to consume increasingly larger quantities of alcohol to achieve the same effects. This third level is called a heavy drinker. The person at this level can consume enormous amounts of alcohol without becoming dizzy. He feels proud of himself for being able to tolerate large quantities of alcohol. The line between the two levels, knowing where one has ended and the other begins, is very thin.

Carmen: Thank you, Sandro, for your time. Everything makes sense. Now I need to put it into practice and live it instead of only understanding it. All I need to do is develop good habits that contribute positively to my life, like a bank account. I need to invest for the future and continue saving instead of withdrawing from my account. Worry about my present, stop thinking about things that I can't control and have a positive outlook on those events. And have faith in a supernatural being.

I like the attachment, and I think I'm a relief drinker. I don't want to go to the next level, and I need to stop it now. Thank you for your help, and have a good day!

Thoughts

One month had passed since I assessed Mary. She was doing well, not judged on the results she was getting but because of the habits she was changing. She was very excited about her life. She said that she was happy, feeling great, eating organic, and eating her breakfast, lunch, and dinner as a habit now. She was exercising by coming to the training sessions and by running on her own. She mentioned that in the beginning it had been difficult to change her habits, but the more she persisted, the easier it got. Mary also mentioned that she did care about the weight she was losing, but the results she was seeing in her life were even more fulfilling: the increased energy, the strength, the positivity, the new supportive friends, and the knowledge and pleasure of making good decisions about her life.

"I'm very happy, Sandro. When you made me sign a contract to stay with your training, I was not sure if I could make it. Now I can see it was the best decision and investment I have done in a while."

"I'm glad to hear that," I responded. "That was the idea, to change your life to a better one."

"I feel more self-confidence," she said, "and there is something about your training and exercise that helps me to think more positively. I don't know if I'm crazy, but I have noticed lately that I have an internal fight going on. I have a voice in my head saying negative things, telling me that I'm useless, that I can't do things, that I feel tired. But when I'm here, I hear your voice, and I overcome those voices in my head."

"I know what you mean," I answered. "Everyone has the good and bad side, positive or negative self-talk. Psychiatrists call extreme cases schizophrenia. But I don't believe in mental disease caused by biology. I believe that mental disease is caused by weakness of the mind. There is an organization called the Citizens Commission on Human Rights International (CCHRI). They are discovering the truth behind the psychiatric diseases. But that is another story."

"So you are telling me that the voices inside me are real?"

"Yes, they are a product of your environment. However, you do have control over your thoughts. What you want to think is up to you. Unfortunately, our brain has been conditioned since we were in our mother's womb. We don't choose our environment, including the family that we are born to. Therefore, we have some beliefs ingrained in our brain that are not actually true," I explained.

"Your brain is like a computer," I said, continuing. "The computer has a hard drive where it stores information. All the information that you have stored in the hardware will lead the computer to perform based on the information. Same thing happens to your brain. All the information, including, *'You can't do that,' 'It is impossible for you,' 'You are fat,' 'You are useless'* is information that controls your brain and your behavior. Society in general contributes to everything you do. If a friend of yours is complaining most of the time and saying, *'This is too difficult,' 'Lifting weights hurts,' 'The economy is bad,'* or *'I hate working in this place,'* you could end up believing it, and it becomes part of you. Another example is television with programs featuring thin women, muscular men, an expensive life, and commercials that equate food with happiness. All these things program you at the subconscious level. Let me explain it in a different way: Your conscious thoughts are like the 10 percent of an iceberg that people can see, and the other 90 percent of your thoughts are covered. You perform on the 90 percent, and that is what gets you were you are. The other 10 percent is superficial."

"You said like a computer, so you can install a program and delete information, right?" Mary asked.

"Yes, you can do that," I answered. However, it does require constantly new positive input and staying away from negative input. One of our members mentors a young girl. The mom of the young girl is an alcoholic, and the family is incredibly dysfunctional. When Melisa comes to meet her mentor, Lorie, she arrives with negative input. Lorie brings Melisa to our training because she wants Melisa to feel another type of atmosphere. Melisa gets all pumped up and ready to start the week with all the input she gets here and from Lorie. However, when she goes back to her family, she struggles again because of the negative input she is getting from her family."

"I see," Mary said. "So I should stop hanging out with negative people. But most of my friends are negative. They complain about their marriage, the economy, their car ...

usually about everything. I don't think a good friend should leave their friends only because of the negative input."

"Have you heard about crab behavior? When fishermen catch crabs, they usually put them in a bucket that has no lid because when one crab tries to escape, another one pulls it back. The same theory applies to humans. We have some crab peers, including family members. They have negative input, and they can pull you back down into the bucket. So, yes, take into consideration all the negative input that you can get rid of, such as crab peers, television, negative news, and gossip. Your friends are not really your friends if they are not helping you succeed. They are pulling you down and not letting you realize your potential. This doesn't mean you should condemn them. They are humans just like us, and you should always hope that they understand they are trapped by their thoughts. But don't try to force them to get out of the trap they have created. They won't do it. You will waste a lot of your energy and get exhausted. When they're ready, they will come to you and ask for help. That is a real friend. You will be there to help them when they want to be helped."

"I think it's hard to leave my friends, and I don't want them to think I don't like them," Mary said. "But I think you're right. I'm usually enthusiastic when I meet with them, and by the end of the night, I feel drained. We don't talk about good things in life. They talk about work, their boss, how they want to change their job and things like that, but they don't talk about an action plan. They just complain. But we also talk about the fun things we have done in the past, which I think is what keeps us together."

"Well, you have something in common," I said. "That is why you get along. There is nothing wrong with that. Wolves in a pack have the same goals and share behaviors, and the same is true with a flock of ducks. They share the same goals and behaviors. This is also true with humans. Look around and you will find that people with something in common tend to get along with each other: successful people, runners, people who like to camp, bike, or go shopping and even those who like to do drugs or be in gangs. People are defined by the group with whom they hang out. We subconsciously learn their behaviors. By the end, you decide who you want to be friends with, not forgetting the end result, your goal."

"And if I put everything you're saying together, you're telling me that some of the negative voices I hear and actions I take are because of the people that I hang out with. Is that right?" Mary asked.

"Yes, part of it. There are other factors, such as TV, your past, music, books, and others. In other words, your environment that surrounds you—including your friends—is the cause of your beliefs."

"Okay, let's say that I do stay away from 'crab' people. What would be my next step, so I can stay away from them?

"The next step is to find positive information or input, self-help books, audio books, and positive people, and even the Bible can help you. Just as you believed negative input, you'll start believing the new positive information you're getting, and you'll perform better. Negative or positive information is like a tape in your head that repeats over and over again. People usually are too lazy to control their thoughts, especially negative input. You may not want to control them, and you'll find phrases such come to your mind such as, *I feel tired this morning.* This thought will become an emotion and in turn will affect the way you feel. So if you think you feel tired, your reality is that you are tired. On the other hand, when you start controlling your thoughts, you decide what you want to think, and this will lead you to thinking positively. An example can be, *This morning is amazing, and I feel energetic.* Even though you may not believe that, your body will start an internal fight to meet the requirement of your brain. In other words, if you don't consciously decide what thoughts you want to produce, then some external trigger —friends, TV or other external information—will. You need to be aware of your thoughts and fight all day until it becomes a habit. Another thing you have to keep in mind is that only one thought can be in your brain at a time. Therefore, when you're thinking about being energetic you can't be thinking about being tired."

"That is the reason I feel good when I'm here," Mary said. "You feed my brain with all your positive input."

"Yes, and you have the ability to control your thoughts, continue feeding your brain positive information, and do what is in your control to avoid negative information. You will feel like you can conquer the world anytime, anywhere," I said with a smile.

"What happens if I don't want to control my thoughts, and I let the negative thoughts control me?" Mary asked.

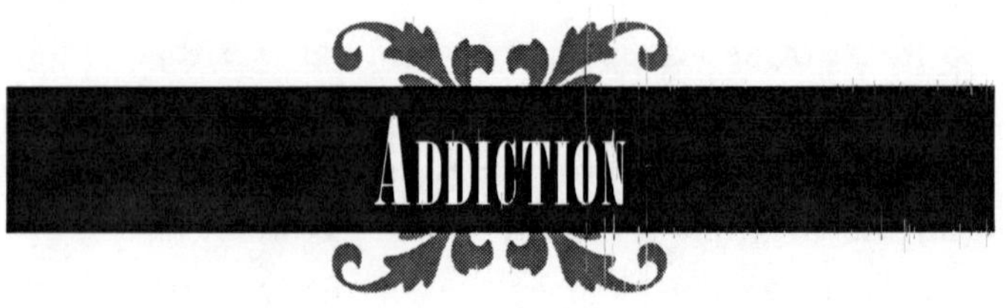

Addiction

"Addiction occurs when people can't control their thoughts and are under stress. Your negative thoughts become desires. What happens when a rational person feels stressed, depressed, or angry?" I asked.

"They look for ways to feel better, right?" Mary said.

"Yes, and when do they want to feel better?"

"As soon as possible would be my guess," she said.

"You're right. What kind of relief do people look for when they can't control what they're thinking?"

"I'm not sure."

"Think about your friends or co-workers or other people who look for prompt relief," I said.

"My friends usually drink when they're stressed. My cousin goes shopping when she feels depressed, and one of my coworkers yells and throws things around when he's angry."

"Have you thought about the consequences of their behavior?" I asked.

"No, but now that you mention it, I'm thinking that my friends drink a lot," she answered. "They start talking about their frustrations, and as the night goes on they start forgetting about it. They spend a good amount of money on alcohol, and the next day they usually don't have the energy to work, and their complaints start again. This has become a routine for them. My cousin is depressed often, so she likes to go buy clothing and things for the house that she doesn't need. She has more than 100 pairs of shoes, and she still buys more, as if she doesn't have any. She said that shopping helps her forget what makes her depressed, which is her divorce and the loss of her son in a car accident. She owes thousands of dollars on credit cards, and she doesn't care, and I know someday she will need to face all the debt. My coworker says that he can't deal with things that don't come out the way they're supposed to. He says he's about to lose his job because of us. He thinks we don't do things according to protocol. What I think is that he wants things one way, and he is about to lose his job not because of his poor management but because of his temperament. Honestly, I think he is a good manager except for how he reacts when things don't go according to his plan."

"These are people who can't control their thoughts," I said. "Most likely, they have become dependent on their behavior or substance without knowing it. Their behaviors or the substance they are taking help them repressed their thoughts. However, those thoughts continue in their head after the relief from the behavior and the substance is gone. This is the reason why they repeat their behavior or substance use. This is called addiction."

I checked my agenda to see if I had another assessment scheduled after her. My agenda was clear for at least one more hour, so I continued talking.

"Let me explain further. It is important to define addiction to understand how an individual may become dependent on substances or behaviors. Addiction has been defined as physical and psychological dependence on psychoactive substances that cross the blood/brain barrier once ingested, temporarily altering the chemical milieu of the brain. Moreover, addiction can also be viewed as a continued involvement with a substance or activity despite the negative consequences associated with it. Gabor Mate is a Vancouver physician and worldwide bestselling author who specializes in the study and treatment of addiction and is widely recognized for his unique perspective on attention deficit disorder. He thinks that there is a general myth that drugs in themselves are addictive. If addiction is understood in a broader sense, no drug is by itself addictive. The real problem is what makes people susceptible to addiction. It's really a combination of a susceptible individual and the substance or behavior that makes the person become addicted, not the behavior or substance itself. To find out what makes an individual susceptible, it is necessary to take life experiences into consideration. Research in pregnant rats shows that the offspring are more susceptible to becoming addicted to alcohol and cocaine after they have been put into stress. Moreover, infants of pregnant women who have been stressed show traits that predispose them to addiction. Furthermore, as we see with posttraumatic stress disorder, life's experiences will bring more stress to the individual. In fact, most individuals with posttraumatic stress disorder have an addiction to a substance such as alcohol, antidepressants, or antianxiety medication. Do you see what can happen when someone is not aware of their thoughts and doesn't fight to control them? Thoughts stress you."

"So if I decided not to control my thoughts chances are I could become addicted to a substance or behavior?" Mary asked.

"Yes," I responded, "That is why there are many people who practice destructive behaviors. They think they will only do it once, and before they know it, they have become addicted. Just as you have described your friends, cousin, and coworker, all these addictions or behaviors bring negative consequences to their lives. And just for the record, you can also find people addicted to food, and obesity is a consequence of this behavior."

"But I thought obesity was genetic."

"Let's say you have two horses, one pure blood and the other a mix. The pure-blood horse is bought by a family who doesn't know anything about horses, and they only want it as an expensive pet. The mix is adopted by highly knowledgeable horse trainers. The pure blood mostly just walks around the stable and isn't training, while the mix is being trained to race and jump obstacles. Which one do you think would perform better?" I asked.

"It is obvious—the one that is being trained," Mary answered.

"While the pure blood has a tremendous potential to be the best in racing and clearing obstacles, its environment is not helping it reach its potential. On the other hand, the mix's environment with the training is helping it reach its full potential. I will explain it to you in a different way."

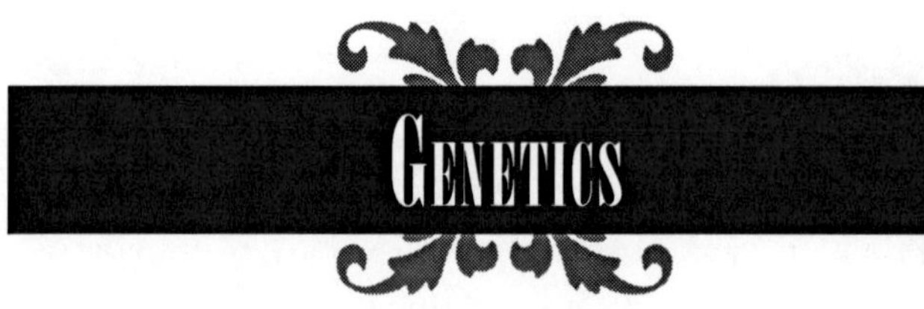

Genetics

"Obesity has been proven to be a predisposition," I told Mary. "A predisposition is a component of the genetic makeup that responds to the environment. When people say 'it's genetic,' they usually think people are ruled by their genes and there is nothing they can do to overcome their destiny. For modern scientists, 'genetic' means a response or contribution from the gene to the environment that the gene is being affected by. Here, let me explain it further. Science has two branches that represent the organism, the living system.

One is the genetic theory and the other is the social theory. Some people accept only one side, either genetic or social. But if these scientific approaches are taken into account alone, they don't tell the whole story. The truth comprises both. There have been studies on genes that have led people to misleading conclusions, such as disease and behavior being hereditary.

One of those studies is the 'twin study,' which concluded that if both twins develop any behavior or disease, that behavior or disease is passed from the previous generation by genes. The only significant problem with this study is that it was performed after the twins were born. In other words, in such a study there is no research on how the environment affects the embryos in the mother's womb. However, in modern genetics, there are many prenatal studies leading to gene predispositions, not predeterminations that clarify the inaccurate conclusion of the 'twin study.' According to Dr. Gabor Mate, 'Most complex conditions might have a predisposition that has a genetic component, but a predisposition is not the same as a predetermination.'

What this means is that genes are not causative and can be shaped by the environment. People who do not know about modern genetics believe 'everything is genetic.' To be more specific, people think that behaviors like eating binges, anorexia, and bulimia are genetically programmed. Genes don't make us behave in a specific way regardless of our environment. Genes give us diverse ways of responding to the environment. According to Richard Wilkinson, professor emeritus of social epidemiology at the University of Nottingham, 'Some early childhood influences and the kind of child rearing affect gene expression, turning on and off different genes to put the person on a different development track that suits the kind of world the person has got to deal with.' Self-fulfilling prophesy can explain the old genetic argument, because people live in the environment that will create the behavior or disease—which is the reason the disease or behavior becomes assured.

According to Mate, 'The genetic argument allows society the luxury of ignoring past and present history, social factors, and economical and political factors that underlie many troublesome behaviors.' When a person says 'it's in his genes,' it is an unacceptable phrase. What the person is trying to say is that there is a genetic contribution to how the organism responds to the environment; genes respond to the environment as necessary to survive. And believing in the theory that it is genetic can be dangerous because you may think there's nothing you can do to change your life. In short, taking into account the conditions of society, it's clear that all behaviors can be changed. We have the power to overcome predisposition to obesity, diabetes, or any other disease by controlling our thoughts and environment."

"Thank you," Mary said. "I have learned a lot today."

Our long conversation finally ended. I handed out her results and congratulated her for the hard effort she had made to get good results.

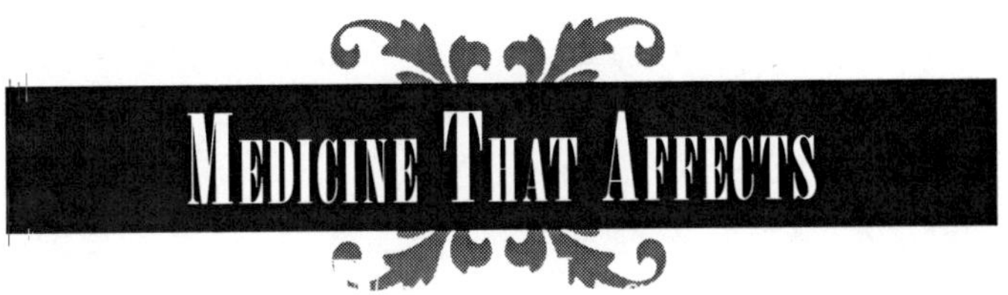

Medicine That Affects

It was one of the warmest mornings of summer. The sun was rising in the east. It was a promising, hot day—one more day at the training studio. People were arriving to their training sessions, and Erick and I were helping them reach their goals. Our day is always perfect despite its imperfections. After one of our sessions was over, Julie came to me asking what I thought about people taking medicine to control some of their health problems. I was not sure why she asked me that question, but I give her my insight anyway. "I think many health problems can be controlled by ways other than medicine," I said. "Nevertheless, many people like the easy way and have become so dependent on medicine that they are not willing to find other sources. Also, for some people it can be deadly to drop their medicine because they are so dependent on it."

"What do you mean?"

"Let's use beta blockers and antidepressants as examples. Many people are not willing to change their diet, exercise patterns, and methods of stress relief to control their blood pressure. Therefore, if they stop taking beta blockers, there can be fatal effects. With antidepressants, many people are not willing to deal with reality. They believe an antidepressant will cure them, but they will need the drug forever. It would be much better if they faced reality and started controlling their thoughts. However, the antidepressant dependent has become so dependent on the drug that suicidal violence thoughts can be devastating."

"But couldn't that hurt them if the medicine is helping them?" Julie asked.

"The medicine isn't helping them in the long term. It's like a pain reliever. If you broke a bone and were given a pain reliever, the medicine would cover the pain, but it wouldn't fix your bone. The same theory applies to other medicines; they cover the problem rather than fix it. Plus, all medicines have side effects that need to be dealt with as well."

"I read something about weight gain with medicine. Can you go to this website and tell me what you think?" Julie asked.

She handed me a piece a paper with the name of the website: *http://www.medicinenet.com/script/main/art.asp?articlekey=56339*

We got interrupted by Erick, who was starting the next session. Julie needed to be ready to go, and I needed to help Erick with the group.

"Okay," I said putting the piece of paper in my pocket.

> *This may be hard to swallow, but a medication your doctor prescribed could be to blame. Certain prescription drugs used to treat mood disorders, seizures, migraines, diabetes, and even high blood pressure can cause weight gain—sometimes 10 pounds a month. Some steroids, hormone*

replacement therapy, and oral contraceptives can also cause unwanted pounds to creep up on you. (Laino, 2005)

Later that night, I sat in front of my computer. The previous paragraph is part of the article I found on the website Julie had asked me to visit. While I knew that some medicines make people gain weight, I needed to do some research for Julie, so I asked the expert on the topic. I got into the College International Databases and started my research. I read the following:

Proxil: Besides birth defects (Drug update, 2006), attempted suicide (Harris, 2004), and sexual dysfunction (Robb-Nicholson, 2001), Proxil promotes weight gain, according to the database (Esposito, 2012). Zoloft, Elavil and Remeron are also antidepressants that increase weight.

I spent a lot of time in different databases reading about the many negative effects of prescription medicine, lawsuits, studies with animals, and people's testimonials about their family. I also found an article that mentions many drugs that cause weight gain:

Mood-disorder drugs that can add weight include the antipsychotics Clozaril (clozapine), Zyprexa (olanzapine), Risperdal (risperidone) and Seroquel (quetiapine). Lithium, valproic acid (Depakote), and carbamazepine (Tegretol) can also put on the pounds.

Drugs with hormonal effects, such as antipsychotics and steroids, are among the biggest culprits in weight gain.

Drugs like Zyprexa—used in schizophrenia and bipolar disorder—cause weight gain of 20 pounds and upward.

Blood pressure medicines that can cause weight gain include Lopressor (metoprolol), Tenormin (atenolol), Inderal (propranolol), Norvasc (amlodipine), and clonidine (Catapres).

Corticosteroids such as prednisone and methylprednisolone are important for treating conditions like rheumatoid arthritis, asthma, and some types of cancer, but they're notorious for adding weight.

With steroids, you're talking about putting on fat stores.
Diabetes drugs, including oral medications like Actos (pioglitazone) and Amaryl (glimepiride), promote weight gain, as does insulin.

Epilepsy drugs prevent seizures. Some, like carbamazepine and Neurontin (gabapentin), can cause weight gain.

Women taking birth control pills also may be "big gainers." (Esposito, 2012)

My focus was on the medications that contribute to weight gain. I copied all of them down and brought the list to Julie at her next session.

"I found some information about the question you had about medicine," I told Julie.

"Let me see," she said as she was checking the sheet. "There are many pills that affect one's weight."

"Yes," I said, and if you pay close attention to the side effects, you may find more issues, such as all types of cancer development, sexual dysfunction, attempted suicide, Parkinson's disease, dementia, Alzheimer's disease, high blood pressure, internal bleeding, birth defects, thyroid problems, and many others."

"But the side effects are only for a small period of time."

"That is what you believe and others want you to believe. Side effects are adverse effects and they are for as long as you take the medicine—and some are chronic, even though you stopped taking the medication. Your body has a mechanism defense called tolerance. This means that your body will become accustomed to the side effects in a period of time. But that doesn't mean that the side effects are gone."

"So, why do doctors prescribe these medicines?" Julie asked.

"There are many reasons, I believe," I answered. "Some doctors don't really know much. They're only following a textbook, and they think that what a textbook says is fact. Others don't care about the client, but they care about the commission they get from the prescription. Some doctors do care about their clients, but their clients may not be willing to make the effort to change their lifestyle. The only ethical thing the doctor can do to keep the patient alive is to prescribe these medications."

"What about if I have a disease that needs to be treated, such as depression?"

"That depends on what you call a disease. AIDS is a biological disease that needs to be treated. Diabetes is a developed disease that we create and can be cured by changing one's life habits. Depression is not a biological disease or a mental disease created by a "chemical imbalance." It's a state of mind where someone is unable to control his or her own thoughts. A pill is not going to cure it. My point is that many people do not need medicine. Nevertheless, there are diseases, like AIDS, that I'm not sure can be controlled without medicine. And in some cases people take medicine because they are not willing to work to be healthy. As a matter of fact, many people like to be sick so they don't have to confront reality. By the way, why are you interested in the topic? Are you taking any medication?" I asked.

Julie avoided my question with more questions. "What about birth control? I noticed you have birth control on the list you brought me. Is there anything else I should know?"

"There are many things you should know. I encourage you to do some research, but I will tell you what I know. Birth control usually involves hormones that simulate pregnancy. Sometimes, as with an IUD, there are no hormones, but they still cause hormonal imbalances in the woman's body. This leads to weight gain and other health issues," I explained.

"What do you think about birth control?" Julie asked.

"There are health consequences for a woman using birth control. I was once married for three years, and I loved that woman. We agreed not to use any type of birth control because of the health consequences. She never got pregnant because we took precautions. Nevertheless, this is always going to be a personal decision. I care about my partner, and I'm not going to put her health at risk. Once I found out about all the risks from birth control, I knew it was not worth using it."

"By the way, answering your question about medicine, my friend started gaining weight after she started taking antidepressants. I thought she was gaining weight because of her depression, but now that you mention it, it could be the pill."

"Or it could be both," I said.

"What would be the best thing for my friend to do?" Julie asked.

"How long she has been taking the medication?"

"It has been four months now," she answered.

"Withdrawal from any drug, recreational or prescribed, is a difficult task. There can be fatal consequences, like suicide or hostile behavior towards others—so it is not advised to just stop using the drug. The best thing she can do is stop taking the medicine under the supervision of a competent team who can support her until she rehabs completely. Just keep in mind that she needs to want to leave the drug. If she thinks that the drug is helping her, you are working against what she wants, and your effort to help her will be useless. When an addict doesn't want to stop taking a drug, they won't, no matter how many times you try to help them. The added problem with being addicted to antidepressants or alcohol is it's easy for people to access them because they're completely legal and accepted by society."

"She's my friend, and her weight is a concern to me, but I think the weight problem is only a side effect of other issues she has. I will see what I can do. Thank you."

Julie reminded me of when I got out of my depression. I saw the opportunity to help a lot of people. But I got rejected many times. When people think there is no need for help—even when there is—they won't accept it. This is the meaning of the saying "When the student is ready, the teacher appears." I once needed help, but I rejected many people until I discovered I needed help. There are only two types of people: those who are rehabbing from bad habits and those who don't want to rehab. Many people relapse when they're rehabbing. I now had the idea for my next newsletter, why people relapse and when people are at the greatest risk of relapsing.

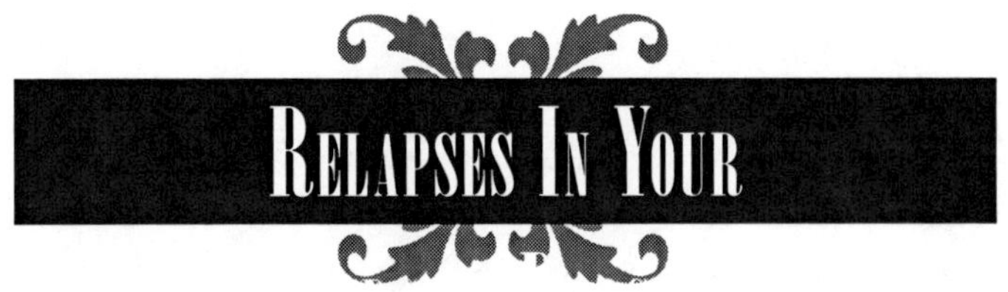

Relapses In Your

I got up early the next morning, ready to write my newsletter of the week.

Resilience: Relapses in Your Fitness Regime

I have some clients that are consistent with their fitness and weight-loss programs: They come on time; they only miss their sessions in emergencies; they keep up their food journal; and they persist year-round. Of course, these clients take vacations and visit relatives over the holidays, but afterwards they come back to their program.

Some of my clients, however, start out with the best of intentions, but essentially they are only in it for the short term and are inconsistent in their fitness and weight-loss efforts. Unlike the first group, they sometimes don't arrive on time to sessions; they clearly don't look forward to being assessed; and they don't keep track of their food. They mean well, but they are not disciplined. Once their contract is finished or even before, they stop coming, but, interestingly, they often return later requesting my services again. And the cycle starts over.

What makes the second group of clients not consistent with their program? The answer is very simple: relapses.

People relapse for many reasons. Stress is the number one reason, but other reasons include injury, illness, finances, and family or addiction issues. Also, among the people who do relapse, some relapse faster than others. People have different attitudes towards adopting new behaviors. This is why people have different levels of relapses, why some individuals are more focused and resilient than others. Psychologists have much to say about this. They call the process of learning new behaviors Stage of Change Model. The stages are divided into five phases: precontemplation, contemplation, preparation, action, and maintenance.

In precontemplation, the individual isn't particularly interested in a new set of behaviors, but he or she is aware that an activity exists. An example is a sedentary person whose friends are also sedentary. They share the same negative habits, so the individual is comfortable with a non-energetic lifestyle. The individual sees his or her lifestyle as reasonably healthy since he or she hasn't really explored other alternatives. The individual may note that a close relative is an active person and seems healthier, but she or she won't weigh the positive effects of taking on a new behavior. I have had interviews with people in this stage. Sometimes a close relative has brought them to see me so I can help them. I've learned that the only effective action that I can take at this stage is to inform them of the negative consequences of a sedentary lifestyle and hope that the idea percolates. Usually the person is not very attentive to what I have to say in such interviews, however. And if someone forces an individual into a weight-loss program, the person will usually relapse since he or she doesn't really care about it. Pressuring an unwilling person into a new behavior doesn't work.

Contemplation is the stage where the individual starts to pay attention to the benefits of a new behavior, but they are not actually ready to change their lifestyle. For instance, the sedentary person begins to notice what the active relative or friend is doing, and observes what benefits they have from exercise, such as having more energy, higher self-esteem, more endurance for physical tasks, and fewer visits to the doctor. The individual may now start to fantasize about having the same benefits as an active peer, but the appeal of their sedentary habits is still stronger than his or her desire to change. To people in this stage, I share information about the long-term effects of inactivity versus how they might begin to feel if they started exercising. The sedentary person often will pay more attention to my words at this point, and he or she will have questions about exactly what kinds of exercise might interest him or her. I figure that they won't sign up for a program yet, but I can tell that they are thinking about it. It takes time for them to get ready; a lot depends on what type of experiences they have and what information they're exposed to. Also, a lot depends on what type of peers they have. If they're in contemplation, they aren't ready to get involved in a weight-loss program; if they get into one, they will probably relapse.

I love to interview people who are in the preparation stage. It gives me energy seeing people who want to progress, who want to change their lives, feel better, and put a stop to many of their destructive behaviors. This is what keeps me motivated. In the preparation stage people are ready to change. They are preparing to enjoy the challenge and results of a new behavior. Most of my clients were in this stage when they first came to me, but they needed someone who could explain them how to break the barriers to self-improvement. In the preparation stage, people want to know the difficulties ahead, to avoid any unpleasant surprises on the journey to acquiring a new behavior. Here people have a high incidence of relapse; they can return to the precontemplation stage due to injuries, boredom, inaccurate information, or unrealistic goals. Because they are only in the preparation stage and not yet enjoying many of the benefits of the new behavior, it is often difficult for them to return to the preparation stage and begin again.

In the action stage, things get more exciting, not only for the individual who is adopting the new behavior but also for any person who wants to see the person succeed in his or her new lifestyle. The individual is now paying attention to his or her food intake and is exercising and looking forward to seeing progress. Assessment is sought after, not feared. Here the person wants to see results as fast as possible. I usually share the testimonials of other clients with them at this point to make them understand that the more effort they put into the program, the better the results will be. Nevertheless, newbies need to be patient and take the program step by step. If their zeal and excitement cause them to want to do everything in the program at once, this may cause overexertion or stress and in fact increases the possibility of relapse.

The last stage is maintenance. The individual has shown discipline to acquire the new behavior. People in this stage diligently work through all the steps of their weight loss program: eating right, showing up at the gym, and keeping their eye on the prize. Even with this success, of course, relapses can happen. But the individual has gotten used to living with the benefits of the new behavior. They notice if they take a few days off that they don't feel as good as they are used to. They've come to understand that no matter what happens in their lives—including additional stress, injury, illness, or even family crises—their new habits will not hinder but actually help them cope with it. Their newfound sense of well-being is a constant reminder of why they are doing what they are doing. Good habits are their own reinforcement to avoid relapses.

Figure out in which stage of change you are. Study yourself, make a plan, put it into action, and try to avoid relapses. If you do relapse, however, just get back on the wagon. Give yourself as many opportunities as you need, and persist in your new habits and behavior. Here are some tools that may help you stay on track, tools that are often more appropriate after you've gotten to the preparation stage. First, get support; get your family and friends involved in your goals. If they are too busy or disinterested, hire a personal trainer who knows how to support you. Make new friends at the gym or in exercise classes who can cheer you along and share your triumphs. Find supporters and confidants who are interested in your new lifestyle. Next, create a manageable diet and exercise schedule and stick to it. Be flexible only in real emergencies. Stay away from places that— and, if possible, from people—who would reinforce your old bad habits. Seek out new activities and people who are part of a healthy lifestyle. Understand that high-risk situations will come along in life where you can't keep up your new habits, but remember that abandoning them will only aggravate any situation. Keep in mind that relapses are not a failure. They are merely a reminder to get back on track. As Publilius Syrus noted over two thousand years ago, "Anyone can hold the helm when the sea is calm."

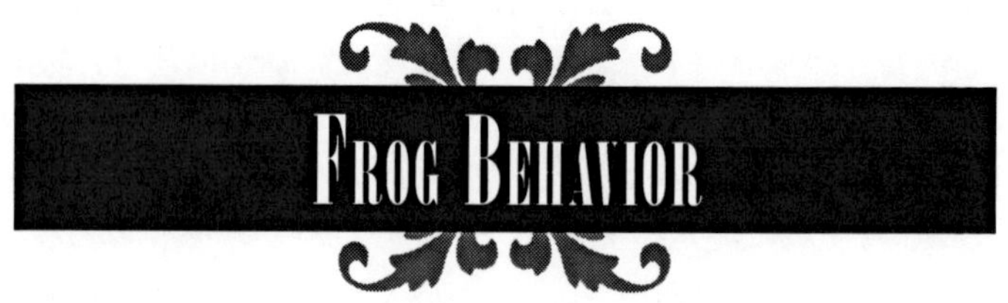

Frog Behavior

It was time to get out there and help people reach their goals. It was another day closer to my goal and my purpose. I had scheduled Mary for her third assessment. She was one of many who were changing their lives for the better. Mary could see the change in her body, but what I was focusing on was her life changes.

"Good to see you," I said, welcoming Mary.

"Good to be here," she said with a smile on her face.

"Are you ready for your assessment?" I asked.

"Yes," she said. "I'm excited to see how much progress I've made."

"Okay, wait for me by the scale, and I will be there with your paperwork. Remember to take your shoes off.

"Okay."

Her measurements were getting smaller—from her weight, skinfold, and circumference to her fat levels. Mary had been a member for four months already, and she had lost twenty-two pounds so far on the scale. When she started, she was obese with a fat level of 38 percent. Now she was at 33 percent, and she also dropped to a fat percentage where she could be measured with the skinfold, which helps measure fat being lost and muscle being gained. The measurements were as follows:

Circumference (inches)	**Skinfold**
Neck: 12.04	Chest: 18
Upper arm: 12.08	Midaxilla: 18
Chest: 36.06	Abdomen: 42
Waist: 29.10	Suprailiac: 38
Abdominal: 33.02	Thigh: 61
Hips: 44.10	Subscapular: 37
Thigh: 28	Triceps: 31
Calf: 15.10	

"You will be proud of me," Mary said, "I've been making a lot of changes. I used to skip all my meals and overeat at night before I started with you. Now I eat all my meals—breakfast, lunch and dinner—and that helps me not to overeat. I have been buying organic, and I stopped drinking. My husband is also aware of the need to eat healthy. It was not easy in the beginning. I'm also more active; besides the three times I come to train with you, I bike, run, and hike at least two times during the week."

"I'm glad you are changing your life and you are enjoying the benefits of a healthy life. I have always been proud of you," I told her.

After four months, I usually take before-and-after testimonial from my clients, and Mary was a good candidate for this.

"Are you ready for your before-and-after?" I asked.

"Not yet, give me more time, I want to look better," she answered.

"Okay, then let me show you your pictures."

Mary stores fat mostly in her hips. She has what many call the pear body. As we went through her pictures—front, profile and back—we stared at her back picture. Her body had gone through a drastic change, and we couldn't believe what we were seeing, especially Mary.

Mary said, "Gross!" in a funny way. "I never realized how badly I was mistreating my body." She got serious as she finished her sentence.

"Do you know that many people do not have an idea how unhealthy their bodies are until they get out of the old frame?" I continued speaking before she could answer me. "That reminds me of when I used to live in Mexico. I'm from the poorest area. There are a lot of gangs, violence, and crime. I saw people shooting other people, guys being beaten into a coma, people doing drugs, and other negative behaviors. I had no idea that I was in the dangerous zone until I got out of that frame. I've read that frogs are cold-blooded animals. They adjust to the temperature of the environment they are in. When a frog is submerged into a pot with room temperature water, and the temperature is increased slowly until boiling, the frog will adjust its temperature until it is too late to escape, and it will die cooked in the pot. Humans and frogs have something in common: we both are accustomed to our environments, and we are both losing our lives in the same way, like the frogs boiling in water. We think we are adapting, even though we are putting ourselves on the burner. We practice negative behaviors, and we don't realize that those behaviors are taking our bodies from us."

"Yes, I know what you mean," Mary said. "I did not recognize myself in this picture. Thank you so much for your help. Doesn't it excite you?"

Since we were still staring at her picture—and Mary is very funny and makes some inappropriate jokes—I replied, "Of course not."

She laughed and replied, "No, I'm talking about the results that your clients get when they come to you."

I laughed with her and replied, "Yes. I have assessed at least four other clients this week, and everyone got good results. This is exactly what we do at Custom Body Fitness. We help our members get results through education, a positive atmosphere, fun programs, empathy, being an expert in body transformation and weight loss, and understanding that we all are human beings and we need support and comprehension."

We set up new goals for her to achieve, and she left the studio very happy because of the results she was getting.

After Mary's assessment, I needed to assess another two members before our noon session. I was feeling confident, and I needed to pass my feelings onto my clients and let them know that weight loss was possible if they wanted it.

The last two assessments were a success. One of our clients lost 2 percent fat, while the other lost 1 percent—not bad for one month. Lisbeth was very into the scale, as many people are. The numbers on the scale meant a lot to her. She weighed 134 before she started exercising with us. Her height was five feet six inches, her fat percentage was 23.2, and she was twenty-seven years of age. In her second assessment she weighed 133.5 with a fat percentage of 21.3. According to the skinfold measurements, she lost seven pounds of fat and gained 6.5 pounds of muscle.

Focus on the Event, Not the Scale

"Why haven't I lost any weight?" Lisbeth asked. "I notice a lot of difference in my body, my brassiere is bigger and my pants are looser, especially at my waist."

"Let me show you something," I responded as I was walking to my office to grab replicas of a pound of fat and muscle to explain the difference. "Do you see this red item?"

"Yes," she responded.

"This is a pound of muscle. Do you see this yellow item?" I asked.

"Ah! Is that fat? Wow, so this is what I have in my body."

"Well, you are doing a good job getting rid of fat. Let me explain it to you. Your body weight is healthy. When you started you fell into the 'fitness' category of the fat chart: You're not obese, and you're close to 'athlete.' This means that you can or cannot lose weight on the scale based on the training you're doing. By that, I mean that if you are doing weight training, you are most likely going to gain muscle. But that does not mean that you are not losing fat. You are putting the same weight on muscle, or even more than the weight of fat you are losing. Many people think having a nice butt or toned arms comes out of nothing, by just doing some cardio. But an athletic body comes from weight lifting.

You define and tone your body by growing muscle, and that helps make a round butt. Your measurements say that you lost 7 pounds of fat and gained 6.5 pounds of muscle, so clearly you haven't lost much weight. But because you're losing the extra fat you notice your body is getting slimmer. If you see these replicas, the pound of fat is bigger than the pound of muscle. Fat is bulkier, even though they weigh the same.

"Oh, I got it," she said. "I think I've been too focused on the scale, you know? Many people focus on the scale, and I think we have the perception that we are going to see results only when the numbers on the scale drop. These assessments are very powerful. If you did not give me this explanation, I might have thought of dropping my program. The mind is very powerful."

"Yes, Lisbeth, this is the reason why assessments are a good idea in a weight-loss program, and you are right. People believe many myths, so it is difficult for them to find reality. The mind is powerful and can blind you from many things when there is no clear explanation."

Lisbeth was happy with the results, and she was ready for her testimonial.

I always exercised at home with workout videos and thought I was pretty fit. But in only three months at CBF I was able to achieve goals I didn't even know I was capable of. I love the group training environment. Everyone is extremely helpful, and we all get excited seeing each other's results. Also, Sandro and Erick are such great trainers. They always make sure we are doing the exercises correctly, and they always push us to be the best we can be. I will absolutely recommend CBF.

I always tell my friends, family, and strangers how amazing CBF is and how quickly I was able to see results on my body and on my health. CBF is challenging and fun. I couldn't be happier with the results. I get so excited every time we do the monthly assessment. The measurements are key for my success. I don't get so busy with the numbers on the scale because they literally don't mean anything. The results will come with hard work. I have lost 7 pounds of fat. But CBF has helped me in so many ways, especially to realize that the number I see on the scale means nothing. The most important thing is to be healthy and happy.

Erick and I started the warm-up. Ten minutes later, our clients were ready to start training. So I told them that I needed to tell them something before we started. I needed to motivate my team. I've noticed when I give a quick, deep speech, our members work out with more enthusiasm. I remember my most recent hike with a friend of mine. I started my speech with a conversation we had.

The other day I was talking to a pretty young lady, and the topic we were discussing was self-confidence. Many people lack self-confidence. The reality is that self-confidence is part of us; we always have it. It is also true that we lose self-confidence during our life's journey. This is due to many factors such as: negative input from our parents, peers, teachers or others; people preventing us from trying new things; the fear of getting hurt; our perception that other people are smarter, stronger, and better than us; and perhaps our fear of failure. The reality is that we can achieve anything we want if we work at it. It's okay to get hurt every once in a while (how did you learn that fire burns?). People are not smarter, stronger, and better than we are, and failures are nothing more than lessons teaching us to try again in a different way. Failures are part of success. They come attached.

After our conversation, I meditate on some factors of self-confidence. As I mentioned, we are born with confidence, but it becomes blurry as we grow. One thing I've noticed we can do to regain our confidence is to break our limitations, get out of comfort zones, and achieve some small successes. Confront the small failures and be persistent. It's just like learning how to ride a bike. It's okay to fall many times, but don't give up until you learn to stay upright. If you give up before then, you'll lose some self-confidence. Maybe you won't feel confident when you are falling and you'll feel dumb. But if you persist, you'll learn how to ride that bike; and guess what? You'll feel confident. This persistence is applicable to all areas of life, including weight loss. That feeling of success helps us regain our confidence. Without getting out of our comfort zone, we can't enjoy the priceless feeling of self-confidence.

You must trust and believe in yourself to be able to get to your goal. The road to a better life is not easy, but it is easier than paying the consequences of not applying yourself. Being lazy has many unpleasant results, such as disease, undesired body appearance, lack of energy, and accelerated aging. On the other hand, being mentally and physically active prevents and controls diseases, gives us better body appearance, results in increased energy, and slows down aging. Nevertheless, only people who believe that they can start and continue a healthy lifestyle are be able to enjoy its benefits.

Here are some affirmations for you to help improve your confidence:

1. *I know I have the capacity to achieve my weight-loss goal. Therefore, I demand from myself perseverance until I reach my goal. I'm starting now!*
2. *I know all thoughts become real and influence my life. I will spend thirty minutes a day thinking about my future life and self and act toward achieving them.*
3. *I know that any thought input will contribute to my daily decisions and will give me commensurate results. I will find positive resources to feed myself with positive input.*
4. *I have written down my fitness and health goals clearly, and I will never stop working toward my desired goals.*
5. *I understand that what I put into the world is what I will get out of it. Because I'm working on becoming a better person, I will help others get to their goals as well. Everyone around me has his or her own fight. I will not judge nor be envious or jealous of others for their achievements. I will do everything with love. I know that a negative attitude toward others will never help me to be successful in my goals.*
6. *I will make everyone believe in me, because I believe in them and, seeing that, they will believe in me.*
7. *It is important that I do not ignore these words but instead that I put these intentions into practice. I will say and repeat these words every day until I have them memorized.*

These affirmations will increase your self-confidence. I recommend that you say them out loud. Your brain is an amazing organ, and it will believe what you feed it. Make one of your goals this year be feeding positive information to your brain. It's a priceless investment. This way, you will lose the weight you've been trying to. Self-confidence is what you need to get to your goal.

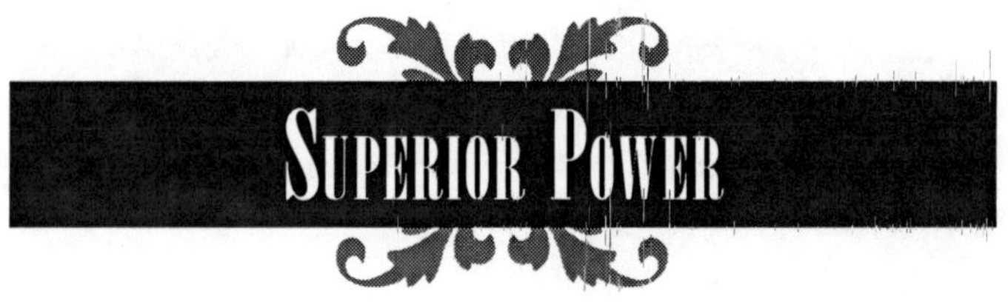

Superior Power

Mary continues losing weight. She is one of the many clients who are still fighting their bad habits. The reality is that many people quit or regain the weight they lose. Marriages, alcohol rehabilitation, drugs rehabilitation, running a business, freedom, and weight loss have something in common: only a small number of people can make them work, usually less than 1 percent. Why? I think there are many reasons, but I will sum it up with two words: commitment and God. People don't have a burning desire to change. They don't want it badly enough. They think they want it, but inside of them, they don't want to pay the price. They want an easy way out. They are not committed to their goals—just like with marriage, where many are getting divorced, making excuses such as *she's not for me*, *it's not the time*, *I'm not in love anymore*, or *we are going to a different place*. People are no longer committed to fight for their loved ones. Love is not a feeling; love is responsibility and commitment. When a person is suffering from drug withdrawal, it is easy for the person to give up like a spoiled child and go back to the drug to stop the pain. These people are not committed to leave their past and pains behind. They prefer to live under the drug's effects. The same thing happens with weight loss. People are not responsible for their actions and do not want to be married forever to their new positive habits. They want to have the opportunity to divorce them, and when they are in pain, it's easy to go back to the bad habit that gives them relief from their pain.

I have noticed a pattern among people who have achieved their goals and are genuinely happy. They have found a path that people who struggle have not. They have found God. God is not a powerful being who rules the world. God is not a king who punished people; God is not a religious image. God is the entire positive action and thinink, a power that helps you overcome everything in life. God is all the good habits, love, responsibility, belief, justice, work, trust, life, commitment, joy, peace, empathy, comprehension, knowledge, nobility, patience, passion, discipline, dedication, awareness, clarity … God is a verb, movement. All the antonyms of these words push away from God.

When we have given our life to God, there is nothing that can stop us. We can achieve anything we want. This is one of the reasons that people who have given their lives to a Superior Power will succeed in their rehab. In fact, we are all rehabbing, and people who are protected by a superior power are unlikely to relapse.

My job is not to sell religion. Religions are beliefs that have been set up by humans. Just as with any organization, religions are run by people, and you will find good leaders and distorted leaders. The best thing you can do is find the best leaders to help you be independent, so you can become a leader as well. However, Mother Teresa said, "A Christian must be a good Christian, a Muslim must be a good Muslim, and a Hindu must be a good Hindu." Religion does not matter. We all are following the same God, and when someone is representing God, it doesn't matter what religion he or she practices.

Take Control of Your Life

Today you wake up after a night's sleep. You must wonder what the day will bring for you. Since past days have brought frustration, perhaps you may think that this new day will do the same.

Now wait a second; hold your thought and rewind it. Today is a new day; you are the creator of your consequences. This time your day is different. Why? Because you know you are responsible for what this day will bring you. From today forward, you take ownership of your destiny. Your days are magnificent. Each week, month, year, and decade are bringing self-fulfillment. Today you have decided to do all it takes to make your day the best day. You are controlling all you can control, such as your thoughts and habits, and you are not letting things you can't control affect you, such as others people's decisions or the weather. You find and look for the best in life, in a rainy day, in a tragedy. Each tragedy brings a handful of opportunities. You give thanks and enjoy all the small things in life. You are paying the price for all your desires. There are obstacles in the way, but you continue to be persistent until you get what you are looking for. You may change the route, but you are not changing your mind about your goal. You have a burning desire to reach it, and you are sacrificing everything you have to get it, except your human relationships, your health, and your integrity. Each day is a step closer to your goal, and you continue stepping even though you have done thirty thousand steps and your body no longer wants to do it. As long as you live, you are standing strong for your dreams. You are not getting distracted by human pleasures. These habits will only delay your dreams. However, you are fulfilling your heart and living a life of transcendence. You know you are a special human being and you are powerful in the hands of a Superior Power. You are given what it takes every day to smile and to make people feel special. You do this because you want to be treated the same way, and love is reciprocated. You think all the time that all you do is easy even though it's not; you make it easy. You forgive yourself and forgive others. You learn from your meditations, from your mistakes, and from the mistakes of others. You set free the aggressors of your life and don't let them hurt you again because they don't have any control over you. By the end—when you turn back and see all the obstacles you have overcome, all the wrong and right decisions you have made, the people you have helped, people who have helped you, the positive changes you have made in this world and people, the people whose lives you have changed because of your smile and all the dreams you have accomplished—you realize that your happiness is in your journey, and all you are accomplishing is only the fruit that you have created, and thankfully you return it to the world.

Today you are exercising like never before, you feel the burn in your muscles, and your heart rate is going fast. An adrenaline rush goes through your body, and you get excited because you know you are doing something to change your body to a more efficient, powerful machine. You meticulously choose the right foods because you know your machine will perform only as well as the energy you are giving to it. Your brain, the computer that runs this machine, is the most powerful organ you have, and you know that. Therefore, you take care of it by programing it with positive thoughts and positive information, and you reset it every day by giving it some quiet time. You make your day better because you decide that today is the day when all the bad habits no longer have space in your life. You have decided to be independent of the destructive habits. Your stress relief is now coming from all the good things that are positively contributing to your life now and later.

When you feel that you cannot take it anymore, think about all your achievements. Think about the seed that you are planting for your future. Think that less than 1 percent of people achieved their goals, and you are part of the 1 percent. You are special. What can be done today, you are doing it. You have faith. Not an empty faith but a faith that is built in action and in persistence, commitment, dedication, discipline, and passion. You trust a Superior Power, not because you let him do everything for you, but because you know you are doing the right thing, and this power will support you.

Your destiny is on you.

My Health & Fitness Plan

My Health & Fitness Plan

My Health & Fitness Plan

My Health & Fitness Plan

My Health & Fitness Plan

My Health & Fitness Plan

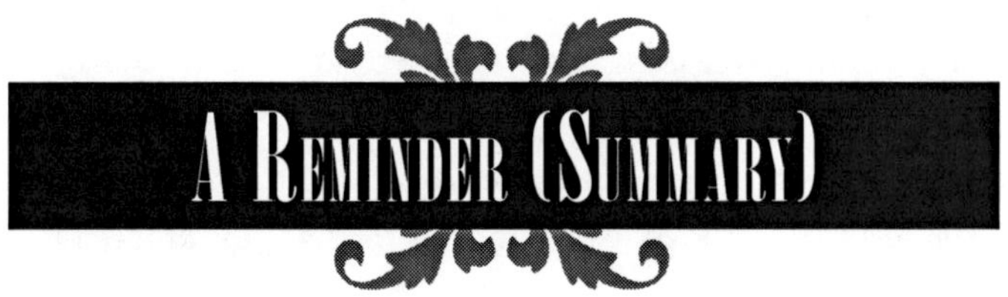

A Reminder (Summary)

In what ways are you different from everyone else?

You wake up early, have a shower, cook breakfast, prepare your lunch with veggies, get your workout in, get to work, have a healthy midmorning snack, focus on work goals, eat lunch, slog away all afternoon, finish the last task at work, and go home. You pick up the kids on the way there, take care of the household chores, cook a good dinner from scratch with the family, and eat with them. Finally, you give yourself twenty minutes alone before bed and choose to read a self-improvement book instead watching TV. Then it's late; you get ready for bed and go to sleep. Even if you're disciplined enough to follow this healthy routine five days a week, perhaps some part of you wants to live a less responsible way: to eat junk food for meals, to stop at the bar after work, to plop onto the couch at home and veg out watching TV instead of reading. But you've tried that before and recall that it didn't contribute positively to in your life, so you stick to your wiser plan.

The good news is the payoff: After a few months of sensible eating and regular exercise, you start to notice a change in your body and your mind too. You feel fit, have more energy, and have gone several months without getting sick. In addition, you breathe better, your back is not in pain anymore, you run around with your kids after work, you feel more alive, and wonderfully you find that *you are losing weight*! How exciting. Also, you are smarter, and your mind is clearer when making decisions. You perform better at work; in fact, people have started coming to you for advice. The healthy habits of exercising, eating healthy, and reading good books are now paying off in your life.

Your family has grown stronger as well. Your strong bonds have deepened with this change of lifestyle.

You feel proud because you know your life makes more sense now. Your life and health goals---some that you made New Year's resolutions—are coming true. It's not like last year when you didn't do it even though you tried. Back then, healthy goals were merely a wish list. But now it's real. You've learned that positive change doesn't happen unless you do something about it, and you *did* do something about it! You've taken your life under control and your quality of life has improved.

This is the reason you are special---because you pay the price of good habits, every day and every hour of your life. You are improving your life, your family's life, and your community overall.

I know you are a leader and can change your life for the better. Something inside of you tells you that you're not alone in this world and that you can change your life because you know you deserve more. This is the reason why you continue reading this book.

I have faith in you, your family has faith in you, and the world has faith in you.

References

Bryant, Cedric. *Personal Training Manual.* San Diego: The American Council on Exercise (ACE), 2003.

Bryant, Cedric. *Lifestyle Weight Management Consultant Manual.* San Diego: The American Council on Exercise (ACE), 2007.

Canella, Daniela Silva, Levy, Renata Bertazzi, Martins, Ana Paula Bortoletto, Claro, Rafael Moreira, Moubarac, Jean-Claude, Baraldi, Larissa Galastri, ... Monteiro, Carlos Augusto. (2014). Ultra-processed Food Products And Obesity In Brazilian Households (2008–2009). *Plos ONE 9 (3)*: e92752. doi:10.1371/journal.pone.0092752.

Canfield, Jack, Hansen, Mark Victor, & Hewett, Les.. *El Poder de Mantenerse Enfocado (The Power of Focus).* Deerfield Beach, FL: Health Communications, Inc. (HCI), 2000.

Center for Wellness without Borders, University of Houston. (n.d.). "The 3 somatotypes," http://www.uh.edu/fitness/comm_educators/3_somatotypesNEW.htm.

Conspirafied0.. "Genetically modified food cause tumors and severe organ damage in rats." (September 21, 2012) https://www.youtube.com/watch?v=z55d_bH0450.

Drug update. Second study links Paxil to birth defects. Rn [0033-7021] yr: 2006 vol: 69 iss:2 -[70]. CINAHL Plus with Full Text. http://sfx-44nhss.hosted.exlibrisgroup.com/44nhss?issn=00337021&isbn=&volume=69&issue=2&pages=[70]&date=2006&doi=&atitle=Drug%20update.%20Second%20study%20links%20Paxil%20to%20birth%20defects.&aulast=&rft.jtitle=RN

Esposito, Lisa. "Prescription meds can put on unwanted pounds." *HealthDay Consumer News Service.* (March 2, 2012) http://consumer.healthday.com/cardiovascular-and-health-information-20/heart-attack-drug-news-364/prescription-meds-can-put-on-unwanted-pounds-662122.html

Fahey, T. D. "Adaptation to exercise: Progressive resistance exercise." *Encyclopedia of Sports Medicine and Science.* Internet Society for Sport Science. (1998), http://www.sportsci.org/encyc/adaptex/adaptex.html

Harris, Gardiner. "Antidepressants restudied for relation to child suicide." *The New York Times*, (June 20, 2004), http://www.nytimes.com/2004/06/20/national/20depress.html.

Hruska, Bryce and Eve Eledjeski. "Alcohol Use Disorder History Moderates the Relationship between Avoidance Coping and Posttraumatic Stress Symptoms." *Psychology of Addictive Behaviors, 25 (3)*, (2011): 405–414.

Joseph, Peter. (director & writer). *Zeitgeist. Moving Forward* [Motion picture; Documentary]. United States: Gentle Machine Productions, 2011.

Laino, Charlene. "Is Your Medicine Cabinet Making You Fat?" *MedicineNet.com*, (October 17, 2005) http://www.medicinenet.com/script/main/art.asp?articlekey=56339.

Lin, W-T., Huang, H-L., Huang, M-C., Chan T-F., Ciou, S-Y., Lee, C-Y., … Lee, C-H. "Effects on uric acid, body mass index and blood pressure in adolescents of consuming beverages sweetened with high-fructose corn syrup." *International Journal of Obesity, 37,* 532–539 (2012).

Lopez, Lauren. "5 reasons people fail to lose weight in the New Year." *Healthy Living*, (December 30, 2010) http://www.examiner.com/article/5-reasons-people-fail-to-lose-weight-the-new-year

McGraw, Phil. *The Ultimate Weight Solution: The 7 Keys to Weight Loss Freedom*. New York: Free Press, 2003.

Meyer, Joyce. *Power Thoughts: 12 Strategies to Win the Battle of the Mind*. New York: Hachette Book Group, Inc., 2010.

Nolen-Hoeksema, Susan. *Abnormal Psychology* (5th ed.). New York: McGraw-Hill Higher Education (2011).

Omichinski, Linda. *Nondiet Weight Management: A Lifestyle Approach to Health & Fitness*. McLean, VA: Nutrition Dimension/Gannett Education, Inc., 2010.

Osborne, Kate. "Hormones in meat: Science or spin?" *Australasian Science 32, (4)*, (2011): 22–24.

Robb-Nicholson, C. "By the way, doctor. I've been taking Paxil for depression for about six months. Although it's helped my symptoms of depression, I've lost interest in sex. Aside from stopping the medication, is there any way to regain my sexual function?" *Harvard Women's Health Watch 8, (6): 7,* (February 8, 2001) http://www.ncbi.nlm.nih.gov/pubmed/11175469.

Robbins, Anthony. *Unlimited Power.* New York: Ballantine Books, 1987.

Sánchez, Carlos Cuauhtémoc. *Los Ojos de Mi Princesa (The Eyes of My Princess).* Tlalnepantla, Estado de Mexico: Grupo Editorial Diamante, 2004.

Sánchez, Carlos Cuauhtémoc. *Volar Sobre el Pantano (To Fly Over the Swamp).* Tlalnepantla, Estado de Mexico: Grupo Editorial Diamante, 2004.

Sánchez, Carlos Cuauhtémoc. *Los fantasmas del Espejo (The Ghosts in the Mirror).* Tlalnepantla, Estado de Mexico: Grupo Editorial Diamante, 2008.

Schulz, Laura C. "The Dutch Hunger Winter and the developmental origins of health and disease." *Proceeding of the National Academy of Sciences, 107, (39),* (2010): 16757–16758.

Sharecare.com. (n.d.). "How much testosterone do women have, compared to men?" http://www.sharecare.com/health/endocrine-system/how-much-testosterone-in-women

Sharma, Robin. *The Monk Who Sold His Ferrari: A Fable About Fulfilling Your Dreams and Reaching Your Destiny.* New York: HaperCollins Publishers Inc., 1997.

The RSA. (2013, September 4). *How cooking can change your life – Michael Pollan* [Video file]. https://www.youtube.com/watch?v=TX7kwfE3cJQ.

Tunick, Barbara. "Does eating meat make people fat?" *Vegetarian Times, 327*, 95 (January, 2005) http://www.vegetariantimes.com/article/does-eating-meat-make-people-fat/.

CPSIA information can be obtained
at www.ICGtesting.com
Printed in the USA
FSOW01n2303100915
10946FS